D0351537

CONTENTS

CHAPTER TWELVE: YOUNG PEOPLE

Honesty. Daily diary. Contracts. Activities. School. University. The future. Summary.

CHAPTER THIRTEEN: ALTERNATIVE MEDICINE 183

Historic treatments (Homeopathy, acupuncture, spiritual healing). Unwind techniques (meditation, massage, T'ai Chi, self-hypnosis). Food medicine (herbalism, folk medicine, Royal Jelly, Probiotics). Detoxification techniques (dental amalgam, colonic lavage). Recent treatments (TEN, sound waves, colour therapy). Summary.

CHAPTER FOURTEEN: MANAGEMENT 202

Medical Knowledge: Cognitive Behaviour Therapy, Graded Exercise. Doctor's role: Medical assessment (diagnosis, other diagnoses, identify patients' problems), treatment (encourage patients to help themselves, support the patient, self-help groups). Patient's role: the media, personal responsibility, finding answers. Conclusion. Summary.

CHAPTER FIFTEEN: CONCLUSION 228

Future medical treatment. A great opportunity. Advantages.

INDEX 235

ABOUT THE AUTHOR

Dr Darrel Ho-Yen was born in Guyana, South America, but finished his schooling in London. After a year's Voluntary Services Overseas in the Caribbean, he went to Dundee University medical school. He completed his training at the Regional Virus Laboratory, Ruchill Hospital, Glasgow. He is now Head of Microbiology at Raigmore Hospital, Inverness; Director of the Scottish Toxoplasma Reference Laboratory; and Honorary Clinical Senior Lecturer at Aberdeen University.

Dr Ho-Yen has had extensive experience in managing and counselling patients with Post Viral Fatigue Syndrome and the first edition of this book (1985) was the first book on this subject. He has written many other books: co-author of **"Diseases of Infection"** (1987, 1993) and co-editor of **"Human Toxoplasmosis"** (1992), both published by Oxford University Press; co-author of **"Ticks"**, Mercat Press (1998); and co-editor of **"Science of Laboratory Diagnosis"**, ISIS Medical (1998).

His experience on the needs of patients with chronic illnesses prompted him to write **"Unwind! Understand and control life be better!!"** (deals with relaxation and stress management techniques) in 1991 (reprinted in 1994) and **"Climbing Out of the Pit of Life"** (deals with recovering from great loss) in 1995. Dr Ho-Yen has published numerous scientific papers and articles for medical practitioners and the general public, and lectures extensively.

PREFACE

The first edition of this book was printed in April, 1985. It was in response to numerous requests from patients and doctors for information on the Post Viral Fatigue Syndrome/Myalgic Encephalomyelitis (PVFS/ME). **I had found that patients needed much support and that hours could be spent on the telephone (at great cost) or in consultation.** At these times I often found myself repeating what I had said before, so it seemed logical to write down my approach and opinions. I hoped that this would allow **patients to read a particularly relevant section several times as patients are often making the same mistakes.**

The first edition of this book was the first book published in the world on PVFS/ME. Since then there have been some 30 books. Many of these books are highly scientific and have many references. However, many patients do not want such precise information, but instead they want more details about my management system. As space in a book is limited, I have taken this advice. In this book, **I have concentrated on what I tell patients when I see them.**

I have been very grateful to the many patients who have been generous enough to comment on the aspects of my book that they have found most helpful. Over the years, I have spoken to very many groups of patients throughout Britain. At these talks, many have felt that my pictorial slides were very useful. **Thus, in this edition I have**

included many of the slides that I use to illustrate my talks.

Each month, I receive hundreds of articles on PVFS/ME research. Each one is an important piece of the jigsaw in this disease, but the important question is: how does this affect patient management now? Each month, I also receive many letters and telephone calls from individuals who have had cures and want to advocate a particular treatment. The question here is: will this work for all patients? At the end of each month, I try to see what changes should be made to my management technique. Over the years, **there have been many significant changes in how a patient is managed.** This has resulted in **this edition being more than 60% different from the third edition.**

This book is designed to be read by ill patients with very poor concentration. The language, type-setting and repetition are necessary. Some healthy individuals may find this style annoying, but I hope that they will understand. As with previous editions, I have received very many helpful comments and encouragement from readers. **Again and again, patients have asked for a book which motivates and sets out a precise plan for recovery.** These have been the main objectives of this book.

No book is published by the efforts of only one person. I am grateful for the support of **Gregory and Colan** during the writing of this book. **Rob Polson** has been exceptionally helpful in getting me scientific papers and proof-reading the many drafts. I have been grateful for help with illustrations from **Alan McGinley, John McGhie, Audrey Grant** and **Seonaid McLaren. Grant Shipcott** of XL Publishing Services has been a tremendous help in typesetting the book, and has managed to meet every deadline. **Forbes Cunningham** of Highland Printers has been extremely cooperative and very easy to work with. Lastly, I am indebted to **Debbie Gilham** who has had the difficult task of providing me with secretarial support; she has done a superb job through the many drafts of this book.

Darrel Ho-Yen
1999

CHAPTER ONE
INTRODUCTION

The whole family was sitting down to dinner. As the meal had been late on the table, all were hungry and busy eating. Suddenly, young Gregory announced that he had dived from the one metre diving board and had been congratulated on his perfect entry into the water. There was no immediate response as all the family continued eating. Then, the youngest son, Colan, remarked:

"So what, Gregory? You said that you did that at last week's swimming lesson".

"Yes" said Gregory, thinking as fast as he could "But actually, last week I was pushed".

This book is written for those who are prepared to dive. It is not for those who want to be pushed. Those who are prepared to be active and do are the ones who will be most helped. As Robert Burns stated, "Let us do or die". Although much has been written about this illness, there is also great confusion. The first difficulty is on deciding on what is the most appropriate name for the illness.

TERMINOLOGY

Many names have been used for this illness:
Epidemic Neuromyasthenia
Iceland disease (1948-9)
Royal Free Disease (1955-8)
Benign myalgic encephalomyelitis
Epidemic myalgic encephalomyelitis
Myalgic encephalomyelitis (ME)
Chronic Fatigue Syndrome
Post Viral Fatigue Syndrome

Epidemic neuromyasthenia was mainly used in America. **Iceland disease** and **Royal Free disease** were terms used after notable outbreaks in these two places. However, for a worldwide illness association with a particular place can be misleading. **Benign myalgic encephalomyelitis** has also been used, but the word "benign" is only appropriate in that there is not a high mortality. It is inappropriate for patients who may have the illness for decades.

Another suggestion has been **epidemic myalgic encephalomyelitis** as this described the occasional epidemic (large groups of patients affected at the same time) form of the disease. However, most cases are probably sporadic (occur in ones and twos as opposed to whole groups), so epidemic is inappropriate. The term **myalgic encephalomyelitis** alone would be more acceptable, and certainly this term with its abbreviation "ME" has been generally used. One criticism of this term is that many patients do not have "myalgia" (muscle pain). In America, the description **Chronic Fatigue Syndrome** has been advocated. This definition requires the exclusion of some 50 conditions and it is possibly less useful. For many patients the illness starts after a viral-like infection, and thus the description **Post Viral Fatigue Syndrome** (PVFS) may be more reasonable. However, a similar clinical picture to PVFS may be occasionally produced by chemicals or other toxins.

I like PVFS as it describes the most common clinical condition and it is an easily understood description. The vast majority of patients remember an initiating viral infection and most patients have previously been well, but one needs to remember the limitations in the use of PVFS. Many have criticised the use of the word "viral" in PVFS as similar illnesses may be caused by infectious agents that are not viruses (such as *Toxoplasma gondii*, or *Borrelia burgdorferi* which causes Lyme disease). However, with PVFS, the "viral" does not imply that all patients have a virus which causes the illness. **Instead, "viral" implies that most patients have a viral-like illness with fever and malaise at the onset.**

INFECTIONS

Everyone has an average 2-7 viral infections every year and these diseases cause over half of the absenteeism from work. The vast majority of people recover from infections within a couple of days, or at the most some weeks (Figure 1). **In the few who do not recover, and who develop PVFS**, the outlook can be bleak. Illness can continue over years, or even decades, and a wide spectrum of complaints can occur. Often, one complaint will linger for months only to be followed with another. Good health appears to be unattainable. **Many**

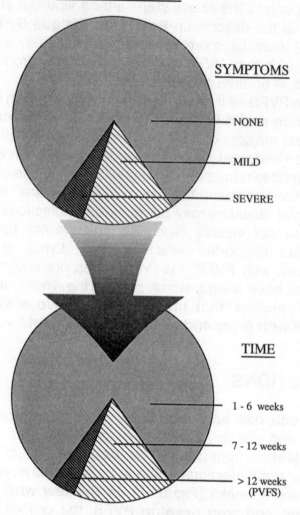

VIRAL INFECTIONS

SYMPTOMS

NONE

MILD

SEVERE

TIME

1 - 6 weeks

7 - 12 weeks

> 12 weeks
(PVFS)

Figure 1 Viral infections and recovery
Almost all of the population have viral infections, and most infections
produce no symptoms. In those with symptoms, recovery in the
majority occurs in 1–6 weeks. A few patients take more than 12 weeks
to recover and develop PVFS.

14

patients become depressed and contemplation of suicide is not uncommon.

Recent medical research shows that PVFS does exist. The suggestion that this illness is "all in the mind" is just not acceptable. Over the last years, there has been a massive increase in knowledge of this illness. Some of the recent discoveries have been due to the application of modern technology, others have been a result of workers in different areas of medicine applying their expertise to PVFS. One can say unequivocally that there is no reason to doubt the truth of many complaints in PVFS patients.

THE DOCTOR'S ROLE

The doctor's role in the management of PVFS patients is critical (Figure 2). He has the responsibility of making a diagnosis, providing information for patients and in motivating them to help themselves. As the illness may last for some years, the doctor will also have to exclude other causes of further symptoms in the patient. All of this will take a considerable amount of time, however, it is likely to result in a relationship of mutual trust and respect. For myself, I can say that a professional relationship can change to one of true friendship. The words of George Washington, the First President of the United States, in a letter of 1783 are as true now as they were then:

"True friendship is a plant of slow growth and must undergo and withstand the shocks of adversity before it is entitled to the appellation."

15

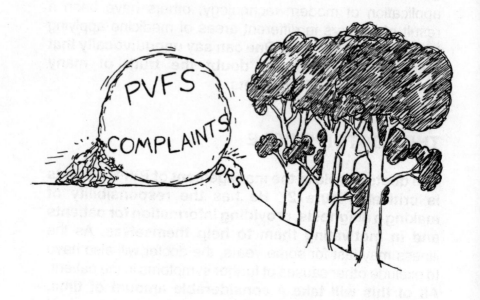

Figure 2 Patients' complaints and doctors
Many patients see the medicinal profession as their major obstacle. In the past this was true, but there has been a gradual change in the attitude of the medical profession. Now, most doctors accept the existence of PVFS.

Loosely interpreted, the relationship between a doctor and a patient with PVFS is likely to be difficult, testing and frustrating; yet as in all relationships, if both parties can try and appreciate the other's position, a true friendship may result.

SUMMARY

1. Everyone usually has 2-7 infections every year, most of which are viral. Quick recovery occurs in the vast majority.

2. For those who do not recover quickly from infections, Post Viral Fatigue Syndrome is the best term. The most popular other names are: benign myalgic encephalomyelitis, epidemic myalgic encephalomyelitis, myalgic encephalomyelitis and chronic fatigue syndrome.

3. Recent medical research has shown that there is no need to doubt the truth of many complaints of patients.

4. The "viral" in PVFS is not meant to suggest that all patients have viruses as the cause of their illness. Instead "virus" refers to the fact that the majority of patients remember a viral-like illness with pyrexia and malaise at the onset of their illness.

5. The doctor has to diagnose the illness, provide patients with information and motivate them.

6. The doctor and patient need to develop a relationship of trust and understanding.

CHAPTER TWO
THE PROBLEM

The scene was idyllic: a sunny day with mother and young son looking at some newly-hatched chickens. The mother was content with life and remarked to her son:

"Look at these young chicks. Isn't nature wonderful? And how do you think these chicks are smart enough to get out of their shells?" Her young son was eager to run off and play football, his immediate answer was:

"Well Mum, they wouldn't have the problem of getting out of their shells if they didn't get in there in the first place".

WHOSE PROBLEM?

In the past, many people looked upon PVFS as a problem which others had, and which the patients could have avoided. However, is it reasonable to say that a chicken would not have the problem of getting out of the egg if it was never in the egg? Of course, it is not reasonable! This is not a question of choice it is more one of destiny. Fortunately, circumstances are changing and perhaps the insight of Karl Marx (1818-1883) can be now applied to PVFS: **"Mankind always sets itself only such**

problems as it can solve".

It is not uncommon to hear: **"I have never felt well since I had the flu a year ago".** Flu (influenza), the common cold and many other viral infections can produce similar symptoms, such as headaches, running noses, coughs, chills and sore eyes. Usually these symptoms clear in a few days or at the most in a few weeks, and then the patient returns to good health. Indeed, many accept and believe in the "24-hour flu" although this concept applies to only a minority of viral infections. **More and more cases are being detected where there is not a quick return to good health.** In these patients, months or years after the acute illness, there are still debilitating symptoms of excessive tiredness and poor recovery after minor activity or stress. In addition, many of these patients have other complaints such as dizziness, difficulty seeing, tremors and pains in different parts of the body. **Are there outbreaks of this disease and how common is it?**

OUTBREAKS

Many accept large outbreaks of PVFS to be:

Los Angeles	(1934)	Athens	(1958)
Switzerland	(1937–39)	London	(1970)
Australia	(1949–51)	West Kilbride	(1980–83)
New York	(1950)	Stirlingshire	(1983)
Middlesex	(1952)	Lake Tahoe	(1985)
Coventry	(1953)		

Many areas of the world have been affected, from North America (Los Angeles, New York, Washington, and

19

Florida) to Europe (Switzerland, Iceland, and Athens) and Australia. **Thus, both temperate and tropical areas have been involved, but most outbreaks have been in temperate countries.** Britain has had many outbreaks (London, 1952, 1964 and 1970; Coventry, 1953; Newcastle upon Tyne, 1959; and West Kilbride, 1980). Four of these outbreaks have been in closed communities; three in hospitals (Middlesex Hospital, a Coventry hospital and the Hospital for Sick Children, Great Ormond Street) and one in a Teacher's Training College. Two of the outbreaks were in general practice and thus both small and large groups, closed and open communities may be affected.

The importance of the sex of the patients has been considered by some to be critical. The hypothesis is that as in some outbreaks women seem to be mainly affected; then, the case for the outbreak being due to hysteria becomes strong, as hysteria is more common in women. Apart from being chauvinistic, this hypothesis does not consider all the available evidence. There are outbreaks that have been confined to army personnel (ultimately "macho"), as in Switzerland in 1937 and 1939.

The most likely explanation of apparent sex difference is that infection spreads more quickly in groups of people: irrespective of the sex of the group, the group becomes infected. **Overall, there are probably more women affected than men, but this difference is not great and certainly not sufficient for "hysteria" to be the explanation of PVFS.** For each outbreak, there is probably only one virus responsible. Virological evidence of Coxsackie viruses was found in the Scottish outbreaks in West Kilbride and Balfron. In the Lake Tahoe outbreak, human herpes virus 6 may have been a co-factor. In the

20

other outbreaks, the diagnosis of PVFS was made clinically and there was no convincing evidence of a viral infection. This is not a criticism, but only a comment that it is very difficult to obtain acceptable virological data. **Thus, patients should not be disillusioned if, in their particular case, there is no evidence of a viral infection.**

I do not believe that the earliest outbreak of PVFS was in 1934. **I believe that PVFS has existed for as long as there have been viral infections – from the very start of man's existence.** Obviously, the limitations of early descriptions depend on documentation. Most cases of PVFS are sporadic (i.e. do not occur in outbreaks) and cases occurring in ones and twos are less likely to be documented. This is an important consideration. Doctors in the past, with fewer journals and fewer doctors, were unlikely to record individual cases or small outbreaks. To be documented, an outbreak had to be large. **Further, centuries ago the expectation of good health was much less.** People expected to be capable of doing less as they got older. People died earlier. Thus, there were fewer cases and individuals accepted their lot as part of growing old.

Therefore, one is more likely to find early descriptions of outbreaks rather than individual cases. **When one goes back into the historical, medical records, I feel that there is good evidence of outbreaks that take us back to the seventeenth century.** The usefulness of this exercise in delving back into history is limited. Yet, there is no doubt that some cannot accept the general hypothesis – PVFS is a rare complication of all viral infections. **Where you have viral epidemics (especially with some viruses), you are going to have greater** numbers (a minor epidemic) of PVFS. For those who cannot accept the general hypothesis, there can be some help and support in evidence of previous outbreaks. This evidence can reassure these individuals that the disease is not new.

ENCEPHALITIS LETHARGICA

What is this? Why is it not heard of now? These are good questions. **Even to the layman, lethargy and sleepiness coupled with disease of the brain (encephalitis lethargica) has some similarity to PVFS.** In addition, there is evidence that the disease occurred in all age groups, but chiefly in the 20-30 age group; social status and occupation played no part in determining those affected. Encephalitis lethargica is probably an early description of severe PVFS.

An early account of encephalitis lethargica was the outbreak in Copenhagen, 1657. Cases of the disease appeared to be related to epidemics of fevers, most likely influenza. After the 1918-1919 pandemic of influenza which killed 20 million people worldwide, a large outbreak of encephalitis lethargica followed. One reason for this is that the influenza strain of 1918-1919 was probably derived from swine. **This particular variant may be neuropathogenic (i.e. particularly likely to attack the nervous system).** When there was widespread vaccination with swine influenza vaccine in the United States in 1976, there were many cases of Guillain-Barré Syndrome (a nervous illness causing paralysis) complicating vaccination. Today, such complications are not seen as swine influenza has been removed from the vaccine.

There have been no large outbreaks of swine influenza since 1918-1919, and coincidentally there have been no outbreaks of encephalitis lethargica. As this swine variant of influenza is much more toxic to the nervous system than other variants of influenza, it produced late complications of Parkinson's disease in many who had encephalitis lethargica. Thus, those with severe illness did not have PVFS or ME as we know it. However, descriptions of those with mild encephalitis lethargica are comparable to descriptions of PVFS. **Descriptions of encephalitis lethargica encompasses the full spectrum of PVFS/ME.** This complication was widespread because the variant of influenza infected so many people. When millions are infected, it is not surprising that thousands may develop a PVFS-like illness.

ARBOVIRAL ENCEPHALITIS

Many arboviruses (viruses that are arthropod-borne i.e. insect transmitted) produce encephalitis. Well-documented complications are fatigue, weakness, drowsiness, inability to concentrate and nervousness. **Some were described as "convalescent-fatigue syndrome".** One epidemic of St Louis encephalitis in 1933 not only shows many similarities to PVFS, but also is instructive on the aftermath of an epidemic. When asked: "Has health been the same, better or worse since the attack of encephalitis?" Responses showed 42% to be the same, 34% to be worse and 24% to be better. **It is perhaps quite revealing to PVFS patients to know that 24% of people can feel better after the illness.**

Other interesting findings of this outbreak were that

mainly adults were involved, and many were incapable of working. Two-thirds of the patients studied were restored to good health with only 7% with total disability. This figure is probably a reasonable indication of the prognosis in PVFS. **Again, the degree of disability can vary with the type of arbovirus, being worse in the winter type as compared with the summer type.**

SPORADIC CASES

One problem with an emphasis on outbreaks is that it can be forgotten that most cases are sporadic. Sporadic cases occur in ones and twos and are the more common presentation of PVFS. At any one time, there may be 10-20 different viruses circulating in the community. PVFS may be a rare complication of any of these viruses. Not all of these viruses can be easily tested for in the laboratory. This is why a diagnosis of a viral infection is often made on the clinical picture. **There is a temptation for patients to blame their doctor for not having the wit to request the correct test.** If there is to be any blame, it is best put at the door of current, medical, virological and immunological investigations. These investigations are not adequate to answer the questions being asked.

A detailed study in the north of Scotland has shown that doctors found PVFS in 1.3 per 1000 of their patients (Figure 3). In this study, 71% of doctors accepted the existence of PVFS. This is a particularly high acceptance rate for Britain, but it means that the figure of 1.3/1000 of the population is probably an under-estimate.

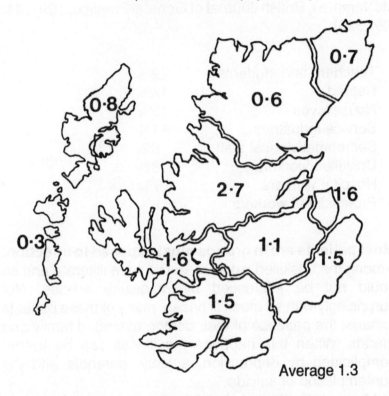

PREVALENCE OF PVFS
(Patients / 1000 population)

0·7

0·6

0·8

2·7

1·6

0·3

1·6

1·1

1·5

1·5

Average 1.3

Figure 3   Prevalence of PVFS in North Scotland
There is more illness in areas of greater population. The prevalence
varies between 0.3 to 2.7 per 1000 of the population. For the whole
area, 1.3/1000 of the population were affected.
(Ho-Yen DO and McNamara I, British Journal of General Practice,
1991; 41:324–326.)

25

PATIENT GROUPS

There is now much more information available on the groups of patients that develop PVFS (Ho-Yen DO, McNamara I. British Journal of General Practice, 1991; 41: 324-326):

Teachers and students	22%
Retired	16%
Housewives	13%
Service industries	11%
Secretarial/clerical staff	9%
Unskilled workers	8%
Hospital workers	7%
Professional workers	5%

Most patients are in groups most exposed to infection. Among the unskilled workers, some were illiterate and so could not be influenced by magazine articles. Not surprisingly with so much ill health, many of these patients exhaust the patience of their doctor, extended family and friends. When this happens the illness can be further complicated by depression, anxiety, paranoia and the contemplation of suicide.

Many patients are hoping for a "cure" from the medical profession. Yet, to many doctors viral infections usually do not last longer than a few months, and hospital laboratories are principally designed to detect viral infections in the first few months of the illness. **Thus, patients feeling unwell years after a viral infection are not catered for by the traditional medical service.** Help for these patients lies in their own ability to understand their illness and to adopt attitudes that change their lifestyle, thus increasing their chances of recovery.

SUMMARY

1. Outbreaks of PVFS have been well documented, but in only a few has a virus been definitely found. Descriptions of outbreaks divert attention from the importance that all viruses may rarely cause PVFS and that most cases are sporadic.

2. The full history of PVFS is unknown. It probably dates back to the start of man's existence. Encephalitis lethargica and arboviral encephalitis are good candidates for early descriptions of PVFS.

3. PVFS is not an uncommon illness, with at least 1.3 per 1000 of the population being affected.

4. In one study, 71% of general practitioners accepted the existence of PVFS. However, for the whole of Britain the figure is lower.

5. Patients need to understand their illness and change their lifestyle to increase their chances of recovery.

CHAPTER THREE

INFECTIONS

Everyone enjoyed laughing at Timothy Dexter. His manners were terrible and his clothes were bizarre. He had left school at eight years and never learnt to spell. But Timothy Dexter had one great gift: he was adept at making money. **It did not matter how ridiculous the project was, if his money was involved, the project was certain to be a financial success.** His rivals complained that he was just lucky, but it was more than luck. Money-making was his destiny.

Timothy Dexter enjoyed other's company although he was always the brunt of their jokes. He listened to his so-called friends. They took advantage of him but he always seemed to triumph. Today, his business ventures would be regarded as the ultimate in lateral thinking. In the eighteenth century, he was an object of ridicule. Most of the laughter was premature. Many who laughed did not care that irrespective of the peculiarity of the venture, the result was always good.

A hoaxer told Dexter that there was a shortage of coal in Newcastle. With his limited education, he did not realise that Tyneside was one of the largest coal producing areas in the world. He bought shiploads of coal and sent them to Newcastle. The story was quickly spread and for weeks it was the most popular joke. **Yet, when the ships arrived in Newcastle, there was a coal strike. Everyone wanted his coal and he made a massive profit.** His so-called friends persuaded him to send warming pans and woollen mittens to the West Indies. Dexter did not realise that a swim suit is sometimes too warm in this tropical paradise. Again, destiny was with the man. His ship's captain was resourceful and sold the warming pans as giant ladles for the large West Indian molasses industry. The woollen mittens were quickly bought by Asian merchants and re-exported to Siberia. Dexter's entry in his diary was perhaps one of great insight:

"I was very lucky in spekkelation".

Despite buying the grandest house in New England and acquiring the English title of "Lord", Dexter was shunned. **No one visited him; no one invited him to dinner.** His snobbish neighbours probably did not appreciate the mettle of the man. At 50 years, he wrote a book which was to become a great oddity of American literature. Entitled: "A Pickle for the Knowing Ones or Plain Truths in a Homespun Dress", it was a sell-out. Although intended to be autobiographical, it was bought for its comedy value. Serious readers had a difficult job as there was little punctuation.

As always, Dexter had a perverse reaction to criticism of his variable writing style. His later editions had an extra page which had nothing on it but punctuation marks. He explained "The Nowing ones complane of my book the first edition had no stops I put in A nuf here and they may pepper and salt it as they please". **Timothy Dexter existed. He was a man who despite those around him managed to live his own life.** PVFS patients must also try to live their own lives despite comments (or even ridicule) from those around them.

VIRAL INFECTIONS

Like Dexter, viral infections are difficult for the public to understand. Viruses are very small agents which produce a variety of illnesses. **They are very much smaller than bacteria and are so small that they cannot be seen through a normal microscope.** To get some idea of the size of a virus is difficult. Nevertheless, a useful simile is that an apple is just as much larger than a virus as Mount Everest (the highest mountain in the world, 29,028 feet) is higher than the apple.

There are thousands of viruses and each year many more are discovered. Some infect animals and plants and others infect human beings. Common diseases that are produced by viruses are measles, rubella (German measles), mumps, influenza, hepatitis A and B, chickenpox and the common cold. **In different countries of the world (especially the tropics), different viruses are found.** The viruses found in different areas of the same country are also not the same. Thus, when a family moves to a new house 100 miles or more from their old house, it is not unusual for them to have more 'colds' and viral illnesses than usual for the next year.

Viruses can only replicate (or multiply) within living cells. This is because they do not have the machinery to produce their own offspring. Instead, they hijack a living cell's machinery and utilise it to produce viral offspring. The whole process is very complex and occurs in all viral infections. **The statement: "just a viral infection" is a** gross underestimation of the sophistication of viral infections.

HOW DO YOU BECOME INFECTED?

Viruses infect the human body in a number of ways. The most common method is through the respiratory tract. A patient (for example with a cold) releases into the atmosphere millions of droplets containing viruses whenever he coughs, sneezes or speaks. **These droplets can enter the nose or mouth of those around him and cause infection.** This route of infection is used by the common cold and influenza viruses and also those causing childhood diseases, such as mumps, measles and rubella. A susceptible person can become infected by shaking the contaminated hands of a patient with any of these infections, and then touching his own nose, eyes or mouth.

Saliva is also a source of infection, especially in respiratory infections. More indirectly, viruses can be passed from one person to another, especially through the conjunctivae in the eyes, by sharing towels or even from swimming pools. Contact with infected animals, especially in the tropics, is another source of viral infection.

An important route of infection is the alimentary tract. In certain patients, especially those with hepatitis A, or Coxsackie infections **the virus multiplies in the alimentary tract and passes into the faeces.** In areas with poor sanitation, these infected faeces may contaminate the drinking water and thus cause widespread infection. **Untreated sewage may be discharged into rivers where they can infect shellfish, such as oysters.** If these shellfish are eaten raw, they can

31

cause infection. As large amounts of virus are excreted in faeces, it is also important that food handlers have high standards of hygiene. If hands are not washed after using the toilet, food may be contaminated and can easily cause infection.

The skin is also an important way by which a virus may enter the body. In patients with cold sores (due to herpes infection), viruses are present in the sores, and thus, contact with these lesions can produce infection. **Penetration of the skin** occurs with bites from bloodsucking insects or animals (for example in the spread of rabies). Drug addicts sharing syringes and needles commonly transmit infection (usually hepatitis B and the HIV/AIDS virus) among themselves.

Although there are many ways for a virus to enter the body, **transmission of viruses from one person to another may not result in infection.** Infection only occurs if there is enough virus, the patient is susceptible and the virus is able to replicate. **If patients have not had a previous infection with a particular virus, they are susceptible, otherwise they are said to be immune.** Unfortunately, there are hundreds of viruses that can cause the common cold, so it is unlikely that anyone can be totally immune to all colds. Whereas, people usually have only one attack of measles, chickenpox or mumps. Artificial immunity to some viruses may be acquired through vaccines.

VIRAL-LIKE INFECTIONS

PVFS can be produced by many infections, but the vast majority are probably caused by viruses. As stated before, the "viral" in PVFS refers to the fact that the vast majority of patients remember a "viral-like" illness at the onset with fever, muscle pain and malaise. There are many causes of viral-like infections (Figure 4).

Although bacterial infections are common causes of infection, Lyme disease and brucellosis are the most important in producing PVFS. **Lyme disease** is caused by *Borrelia burgdorferi* and infection is transmitted by a tick bite. Usually there is a characteristic rash (erythema chronicum migrans) at the site of the bite, and joints may be affected. Treatment is with antibiotics, initially with a tetracycline but later with cefotaxime or ceftriaxone. In individuals in which the diagnosis is difficult, there should be a trial of treatment.

Brucellosis is another important infection which causes PVFS. (*Brucella abortus* from cattle, *B. melitensis* from goats and sheep and *B. suis* from pigs). Infection can be from consumption of unpasteurised milk, or from direct contact with infected tissues especially products of conception. Since the early 1980's brucellosis from unpasteurised milk has been rare in Britain. Infection is common in vets, farmers and abattoir workers. Diagnosis of chronic brucellosis can be difficult and antibiotic treatment is less effective.

Protozoal infections especially toxoplasma may also cause PVFS. The causative organism is *Toxoplasma gondii*. It is estimated that 5% of PVFS is caused by toxoplasma. Infection is acquired directly or indirectly from cat's faeces. Thus, cat litter trays, unwashed vegetables from contaminated soil or sand pits are major sources of infection. Indirect infection may be acquired by consumption of undercooked meat or not washing hands after handling contaminated meat. Infection can be

VIRAL - LIKE INFECTIONS

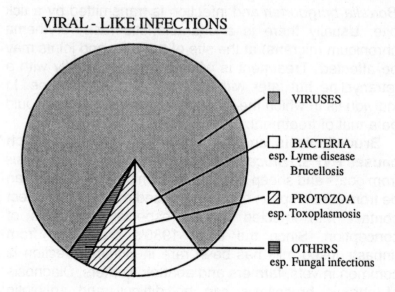

☒ VIRUSES

☐ BACTERIA
esp. Lyme disease
Brucellosis

▨ PROTOZOA
esp. Toxoplasmosis

▤ OTHERS
esp. Fungal infections

Figure 4 Viral-like infections
These are produced mainly by viruses, but also by bacteria and protozoa. Unless specific laboratory investigations are undertaken, it can be difficult to identify specific causes of such illnesses. The attraction of the name PVFS is that it describes the early, clinical illness. PVFS does not mean that viruses are the only cause of the disease.

diagnosed serologically, but antibiotic therapy is only indicated in a small number of patients with chronic toxoplasmosis.

Fungal infections may produce a viral-like illness, and it is possible that some fungal infections may produce PVFS. **Fungal infections probably play a more common role as a secondary complication of PVFS.** Thus, individuals who are ill with PVFS may be more susceptible to fungal infections such as *Candida albicans*. Treatment of such a secondary infection may improve the PVFS but would not cure it.

IMMUNOLOGY

The immune system protects the body against infections. **As any system in the body, it may be normal, less active or too active.** In patients with PVFS, this spectrum of activity can also be found. Some patients complain of developing every infection that is around, and in these patients their immune system may have reduced function. Others complain of never actually developing an infection but feeling as though they are about to have an infection. In these patients, the body's immune system may be activated so that infections do not have time to develop.

The symptoms of PVFS may be produced by two mechanisms: reduced ability of the immune system to deal with infection; or, by the immune system becoming activated after an infection and unable to switch itself off. This latter mechanism is akin to a country prepared for battle, in which all invaders (infections) are rapidly repelled, but the resources of the

35

country are being used up by the army. It is likely that both mechanisms exist at different times of the illness, or in different individuals.

An important group of cells in the body's immune system are the lymphocytes. There are four important sub-populations of lymphocytes: **B lymphocytes** which produce antibodies against specific infections; **T-helper lymphocytes (T-h)** which help other cells to destroy infectious agents; **T-suppressor lymphocytes (T-s)** which stop the body's immune response; and **natural killer cells (NK)** which are the body's first-line of defence against infections.

Lymphocytes and some other cells produce a large group of proteins called **cytokines.** Cytokines control many biological processes throughout the body, but are also critical in the body's immune response. The best characterised cytokines are probably the **interferons** and **interleukins**; these play an important role in the body's defences against infection. Through cytokines, the immune system is able to have effects on all parts of the body and so, for example, can pass through the blood-brain barrier to affect the central nervous system. **Cytokines are also principally responsible for many of the effects of infection such as fever, muscle pain and malaise.** In one study of interferons in PVFS patients, levels of interferons in the blood were not greatly elevated. Nevertheless, it was suggested that cytokines may be mainly acting in affected organs rather than on the whole body (Ho-Yen DO et al Lancet 1988; 1:125).

In PVFS, the immune response appears to vary in different parts of the world. Different causative agents may produce different immune responses. The best explanation of the results is that **in different parts of the**

SEQUENCE of EVENTS

Low NK cells (? consumption)
(more serious illness)

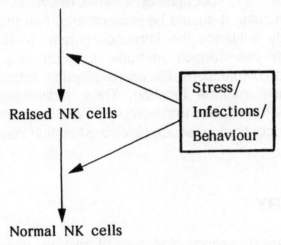

Raised NK cells

Stress/
Infections/
Behaviour

Normal NK cells

Figure 5 Natural Killer cells
It is postulated that there is an initial low NK cell result (probably because of consumption of NK cells fighting the infection or a serious illness); the body responds by producing a raised NK cell result to combat the infection; finally, the NK cell result returns to normal as the body recovers. Progress to subsequent stages is influenced by stress, infections and behaviour.
(Ho-Yen DO et al. Scandinavian Journal of Infectious Diseases 1991; 23:711-716.)

37

world, the major causes of PVFS are different. Worldwide immune responses in PVFS are:

Country	T-h	T-s	NK
America	Raised	Normal	Normal/Reduced
Australia	Reduced	Normal	Normal
Scotland	Normal	Raised	Normal/Raised

The results of the NK cells variations in the Scottish study led the authors to speculate on a series of events (Figure 5) . In particular, it should be remembered that the mind can greatly influence the immune system. Stress and depression can reduce immune function and allow propagation of infections. Excessive physical activity may also reduce immune function. Thus, individuals may predispose themselves to developing PVFS and once they become ill, continuing reduced immune function may delay recovery.

SUMMARY

1. There are thousands of viruses of animals, plants and man, and each year many more are discovered.

2. Viruses can infect a human in many ways, especially through the nose, eyes and mouth.

3. In PVFS, the "viral" refers to "viral-like" illnesses (fever, muscle pain and malaise) which are usually caused by viruses, but also by bacteria, protozoa and fungi.

4. The immune system is responsible for the body's defences. In PVFS, symptoms may be produced by a reduced or increased activity of the immune system.

5. There are worldwide differences in T-helper, T-suppressor and natural killer cells which may be related to different infections causing PVFS in different countries.

6. Immune function may be reduced by stress, depression and excessive physical activity.

CHAPTER FOUR
SYMPTOMS AND DIAGNOSIS

An old, weather-beaten farmer came into the surgery one day to make an appointment for the doctor to see his wife.

"Gladly," said the doctor "Is she ill?"

"Well, I'm not exactly sure, doctor".

"What is she complaining of?" asked the doctor.

"She doesn't really complain, doctor" replied the farmer "But, take yesterday. She got up at 4 o'clock, milked the cows, made breakfast for the family, washed the clothes, cleared the barn, made the month's cheese, cooked lunch, planted the vegetables, weeded the garden, made dinner, did the washing-up and started the sewing. Then, without any warning, at 11 o'clock at night she started saying she felt tired. I think, doctor, that you will have to give her a tonic or something to pick her up".

One person's expectation of good health can be quite different from another. Thus, some feel that they are ill if they cannot do the work of two normal people. Whilst someone else may describe good health as "having no pain". Good health is therefore open to individual interpretation and expectation.

SYMPTOMS

What a patient complains of (his/her symptoms) is a personal, subjective opinion. It is difficult for other people to fully appreciate the severity of the symptoms. "Agonising pain" for one person may be just "uncomfortable" for another. A description of "a tickling sensation in the arms" was so severe for one patient that it was "torture", whereas another patient described the same sensation as "a wonderful, relaxing feeling".

Symptoms of infection such as fever, malaise, muscle pain and tiredness are commonly found either individually or together. **Most such complaints are due to viral infections, but other infections can produce a similar clinical picture.** Any other symptoms that the patient may have influences the doctor to make a diagnosis, for example a scarlet rash is indicative of the bacterial infection of scarlet fever.

Viral infections are complicated as they may be acute, chronic or latent. Acute infections are usually over in a few weeks, and rarely last some months. **Chronic** infections last months or years. **Latent** infections are when the virus remains quiet in the body in between bouts of illness (for example, shingles or cold sores). Symptoms of acute infections are well known: the characteristic rash of chickenpox, measles or rubella; the salivary gland enlargement of mumps; the running nose, cough and fatigue of the common cold or influenza; and the yellow skin (jaundice) of hepatitis A, B and C.

Less well known is that other viruses are common causes of respiratory tract infection, diarrhoea or infection of the nervous system. **Any part of the body can develop a virus infection,** and the medical literature has evidence of viruses producing symptoms in every system of the body.

Generally, most people recover from a viral infection in a few weeks. The recovery is complete and the patient feels as well as he did before the infection. However, in a small number of cases this does not happen. In these patients, the acute infection lasts longer and then the acute symptoms stop, but there is no return to good health. Instead there is a prolonged period of ill health. This results in a number of characteristic conditions of which the most common is probably PVFS.

As PVFS progresses, symptoms may disappear and new symptoms arise. Thus, patients may initially be particularly worried about muscle pain, but after a few years, headaches may be the major complaint. Similarly, a patient may adjust to tiredness but find it quite difficult to come to terms with difficulty in finding the right words (dysphasia). Generally, the longer the illness progresses, the complications become worse. **This is a great incentive for patients to try and get better soon. Sadly, many patients want to get better, but adopt behaviour patterns that make recovery unlikely.**

PVFS

It is likely that many infections, especially viral infections can cause PVFS, however, it is particularly common after certain infections. Thus, **Epstein-Barr virus** which causes infectious mononucleosis (commonly called glandular fever) is characterised by a sore throat, enlargement of the lymph nodes in the neck, a prolonged fever and malaise with fatigue. A popular description of

42

infectious mononucleosis is "the kissing disease", as infection often occurs from transfer of the virus in saliva during a kiss. Hepatitis A is a common infection of tropical countries and visitors can easily become infected; PVFS is a common complication. Hepatitis C is a recently recognised illness which can be particularly debilitating and is a frequent cause of PVFS.

Coxsackie infections do not usually produce any symptoms, but sometimes a variety of syndromes may develop. Acute infection may affect the brain (with headache, vomiting, pain in the eyes when looking at lights, and stiffness of the neck and spine), heart (with severe pains in the left chest) and muscles **(Bornholm disease)**. Bornholm is a Danish island where the disease was first described in 1872. Nearly a quarter of the island's inhabitants developed the illness after attending a wedding feast. One 10 year old boy "suddenly threw himself down on the lawn, screaming" because of the pain in his side. Similar outbreaks **(epidemic myalgia)** have been described all over the world, and in America the disease was called **"devil's grip"** because of the severity of the pain. Coxsackie infection is spread from the faeces of infected persons. **The outlook is good and patients do not die from the disease, although during the illness they may feel that they are about to die.** The acute disease often only lasts a few days, but occasionally persists for a few weeks. In only a very small minority is there persistence of symptoms and development of PVFS.

From the above, it is apparent that many infections are not new diseases. What is new is the recognition that in a minority of patients, PVFS develops. Nevertheless, some doctors, especially those who have been qualified for some time, do not accept its existence

43

and may question the truthfulness of the patient. **Many patients with PVFS are unjustly accused of malingering.**

SYMPTOMS OF PVFS

The age and sex distribution of patients is as in Figure 6. All ages are affected and the male: female sex ratio is approximately the same. For both sexes, there is a difficulty in explaining the double peak at 25-29 years and 40-44 years. What is the reason for these results? Are these two age ranges subjected to particular stress and infection risks? No one knows. I like the theory that at 25-29 years, you recognise that you are not going to live forever; and at 40-44 years, you know that if you make it to 50 years, you will be doing well.

The symptoms of PVFS are many and varied. The most common complaint is fatigue, from which the syndrome derives its name. Other symptoms are best divided into: general, muscular, vascular, neurological, gastrointestinal, cardiac and respiratory. This division is artificial and many symptoms overlap the divisions, for example tiredness is a general symptom but may be related to muscular weakness or neurological anxiety about being tired. Yet, there is some value in looking at the symptoms in the above grouping, especially in patients who have difficulty in understanding what is wrong.

Another common complaint is the feeling of ill-health (malaise). This general complaint is usually accompanied by excessive tiredness and exhaustion. **In some patients their inactivity is accompanied by increased sweating, and worse, well-wishers saying that they should rest**

44

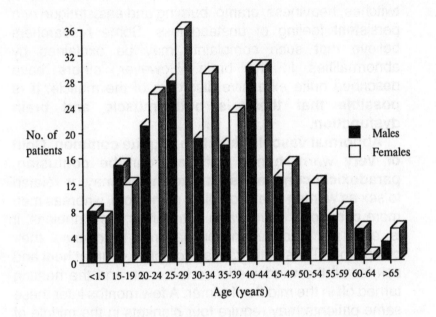

Figure 6 Age distribution of patients
All ages are affected. There is a double peak at 25–29 years and
40–44 years in both sexes. In this study incidence was almost equal
(204F : 177M = 1.2F : 1.0M).
(Ho-Yen DO, Scottish Medical Journal, 1988; 33:368–9.)

more as they were sweating. Explanations by the patient are regarded with disbelief. After all, to the average citizen, one sweats when one is active, anything else is just outside their sphere of understanding.

Muscular problems are present in the majority of patients. There can be muscle pain, weakness, tremors, twitches, heaviness, cramp, burning and easy fatigue or a persistent feeling of unsteadiness. Some researchers believe that such complaints may be explained by abnormalities in the brain. However, others have described quite extensive disorders of the muscle. **It is possible that there is both muscle and brain dysfunction.**

Abnormal vascular function is quite common. Cold or very warm hands and feet can be confusing, paradoxical complaints. An explanation may be related to sex as women often complain of the cold, whereas men more commonly have warm extremities. Nevertheless, it is also not uncommon for patients to change their complaints. Thus patients may complain of great heat and ask for all the windows to be left open and the heating turned off in the middle of winter. A few months later these same patients may require four blankets in the middle of summer because of the cold. Such major changes in attitudes can be particularly difficult for spouses. In both sexes, friends may comment that there is loss of colour in the face. **This could be described as "pallor" or even a "grey, mask-like appearance".**

Neurological symptoms are probably the most diverse, and perhaps the most worrying. Headaches may last several weeks and cause the patient much anxiety. Light-headedness, dizziness, sensitivity to temperature, ringing in the ears, blurred vision and sore

46

eyes are common complaints. Difficulty in speaking or finding the right words, poor memory, tingling in the limbs or loss of sensation in different parts of the body are less common. Fears, depression, poor concentration and contemplation of suicide are much more complex symptoms, but are frequently found.

Gastrointestinal symptoms are very common and in many cases may be related to the development of food intolerance or allergy. A feeling of not being hungry (anorexia) can occur on its own or is sometimes related to patients' frustration with their illness. Not surprisingly, in this group weight loss can be a sequel. Diarrhoea can vary between a few extra stools each day to "streaming, almost like water with a horrible smell" which may occur over ten times a day. **Many complain of alternating diarrhoea and constipation.** Vomiting is very rare and must be distinguished from nausea at the sight of food. Pain in the abdomen and a feeling of abdominal distension is common and may be a result of gastrointestinal muscle dysfunction.

Cardiac and respiratory complaints can be a part of the acute illness. When they persist, as part of PVFS, their severity is much reduced. Pains in the chest, awareness of the heart beating **(palpitations)** and difficulty in breathing **(dyspnoea)** are the usual symptoms. Attacks may not be predictable, but in some patients, particular events or times of the day (especially late at night) are associated with most attacks.

DIAGNOSIS

Ideally the diagnosis of PVFS should be made by a doctor.

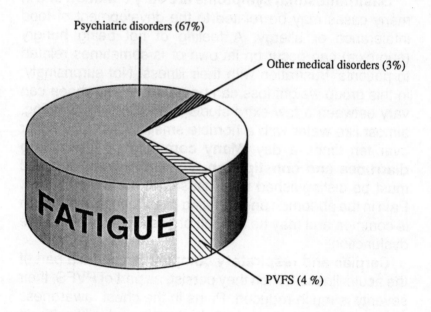

Psychiatric disorders (67%)

Other medical disorders (3%)

FATIGUE

PVFS (4 %)

Figure 7   Fatigue
If only the complaint of fatigue is considered, the majority of patients
(67%) will have a psychiatric disorder. However, if a strict definition
of PVFS is used only about 4% of patients with fatigue will have PVFS.
A small number (3%) will have another medical disorder.

48

Unfortunately, it is wrong to think that the diagnosis could be made in a patient with just fatigue. Fatigue can be caused by many conditions. Indeed, fatigue is a common complaint in patients with psychiatric disorders (Figure 7). This is one of the reasons why some patients with PVFS are believed to have a psychiatric illness.

Diagnostic criteria for PVFS
(Ho-Yen DO. British Journal of General Practice, 1990; 40:37-39)

Definition
The patient with post viral fatigue syndrome:
1. has had generalised, relapsing fatigue exacerbated by minor exercise causing disruption of usual daily activities (at least 50%) for three months.
2. complains of prominent disturbance of concentration and/or short term memory impairment.
3. has no other *obvious*, organic causes for a similar syndrome.

Supporting evidence
(at least four items from sections A, B and C)

A. History
Patient well before illness
An initiating viral illness (clinical description/viral serology)
Myalgia
Gastrointestinal disturbance
Headaches
Depression
Tinnitus

49

Paraesthesiae
Sleep disturbance
Cardiovascular complaints
Adverse effect of alcohol
Adverse effect of heat

B. Clinical
Lymphadenopathy
Localised muscle tenderness
Pharyngitis

C. Laboratory
Evidence of viral infection
Abnormalities in immune function

It is important that the doctor takes a detailed history and makes a full clinical examination. **Several hundred conditions may produce a similar illness and it is the doctor's responsibility to exclude any other cause of the patient's complaints.**

INVESTIGATIONS

Several initial investigations apply to most patients. **There are non-specific changes** which show that the patient has an infection, but there is no indication of the cause of the infection. Secondly, **there are specific changes** indicative of a particular infection. These are usually antibodies which are produced by the body's lymphocytes to help to kill the infecting organism. **Unfortunately, there can be great difficulty in diagnosing viral infections.** Problems often occur in patients who are ill for months or years. Attempts to grow the virus are usually futile because in only a few cases are symptoms due to continuing infection.

In individual patients, it may be appropriate to attempt to identify specific causes of PVFS. A respiratory infection screen and coxsackie neutralisation tests should be done. If tick bites are common, Lyme disease should be excluded. In patients with recurrent sore throats, Epstein-Barr virus infection should be considered. Persisting lymphadenopathy is also a feature of Epstein-Barr virus infection or toxoplasmosis. In patients with abnormal liver function tests, Hepatitis C should be excluded. If facilities are available, it can be useful to demonstrate immunological abnormalities.

The diagnosis of chronic bacterial, protozoal and fungal infections may be equally difficult. Again, investigations may have to be done in specialised laboratories. Often, results are only supportive rather than diagnostic of the condition. Immunological investigations should also be undertaken as these may identify abnormalities.

Any additional medical condition indicated by the patient's history or clinical examination should be excluded. It is also usual to administer a questionnaire to detect any psychological disorder. The Hospital Anxiety and Depression (HAD) questionnaire (Acta Psychiatrica Scandinavica 1983; 67:361-370), or a questionnaire for general medical settings (British Medical Journal 1988; 288:897-900) are both useful.

Before doctors diagnose PVFS, they must consider whether or not there could be other causes of the patient's symptoms. This is not only essential, but also serves to reassure both the patient and the doctor that there is not a more easily treated cause of the patient's complaints. Thus, PVFS is diagnosed by the characteristic history, excluding other causes of the patient's symptoms, and finding immunological or viral evidence of a past infection.

TIME TO RECOVERY

The length of time that symptoms persist is a constant source of anxiety for patients, their relatives and their friends. Most people's experience of a viral disease (and in many cases their doctor's experience) is of an acute illness, lasting at most a few weeks. **Whereas this is absolutely true, equally true is that most people's experiences are very limited.** Anyone prepared to read the medical literature would be convinced, because of the numerous descriptions of individual cases and of outbreaks of illness, that the effects of a viral illness can persist for years. It is reasonable to expect to win the football pools, or to be a national newspaper's millionaire bingo winner. **It is unreasonable to plan your life in the expectation of rapid recovery, or winning a fortune.** Such expectations put a strain on a patient's recovery, and worse when they do not materialise, depression follows. **A superior approach to the problem is to plan a change of lifestyle and a gradual recovery over months or years.** Support from relatives and friends on this basis is much more constructive, and more, such help reinforces any progress that is made.

I find that when patients follow the plan in this book, they recover on average one point every two months. The **very best patients can recover two points in two**

52

months. Most patients that I see take 10-12 months to recover. Often there is good progress until 5/10 and then the patient gets stuck. The patient is often feeling so much better than 1/10 that there is an acceptance of this level of recovery. Next, some patients get stuck at 7/10. If patients can pass 7/10, there is usually complete recovery.

Therefore, **the vast majority of patients recover within the first year.** Of the remainder, most recover within two years. If a patient is ill for a longer time, the chances of recovery progressively decreases. **This is largely because the length of illness is a reflection of a patient's ability to change his/her lifestyle.** The longer that individuals have been trying to do this without success, the less likely are their chances of success. It is similar to passing the driving test. The longer a person has been trying to pass the test, the chances of success becomes less. **Nevertheless, it is possible for patients to recover even after many decades of illness.** Similarly, Mrs Miriam Hargrave passed her driving test at her 40th attempt after 212 lessons when she was aged 62 years.

Why do people find it so difficult to accept that recovery may take years, and that some people may never totally recover? Everyone would understand gradual improvement after a serious car accident. If there is a diagnosis of advanced cancer, any improvement would be looked upon as a miracle. **Attitudes to viral infections are different because there is nothing to see (unlike the car accident), and people's experiences are limited.** They do not realise that some viral infections can have an effect on the body very similar to cancer.

THE SOLUTION

The solution to patients' problems is first to recognise their situation, all patients with PVFS are in vicious circles (Figure 8). A few patients do not recognise that they are in such circles, and many would refuse to consider the possibility that such situations may exist. **The recognition of the existence of these vicious circles is often the key to developing a plan for recovery from PVFS.** A major objective of the plan is to remove patients from vicious circles that make their illness worse.

Many patients with PVFS were high achievers before their illness and one great problem is the lack of achievement that comes with the illness (Figure 8). The isolation of minimal activity, little money, and no social life is difficult to cope with, especially as many patients were previously "the life and soul" of parties. Close relationships, especially sexual ones, undergo tremendous strain. Fortunately, most patients recognise that their current position is one in which they are in vicious circles. However, the difficulty is that **they see no way to extricate themselves from these circles.** The approach of this book is to get patients out of their vicious circles.

Better recovery does not mean immediate recovery. There is **only** slow, gradual recovery from PVFS. What can be learnt is that if life is lived in the same way as before the viral illness, recovery will be even slower. **Instead, a change of lifestyle will allow a better and faster recovery,** especially if the change takes into account the different needs of the body after a viral infection. It is hoped that sufficient information will be provided in this book to enable patients to adopt a positive approach to their

VICIOUS CIRCLES

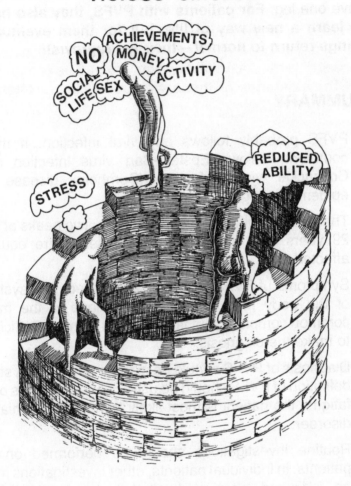

Figure 8
Patients' under-performance in many areas can produce tremendous stress. This stress produces further, reduced performance. Patients extricate themselves from these vicious circles.

55

illness. It is similar but better than having a leg amputated. With one leg , patients have to learn a different approach to life's problems, and eventually hardly notice that they have one leg. **For patients with PVFS, they also have to learn a new way of life, but for them eventually things return to normal – their leg regrows!!**

SUMMARY

1. PVFS probably follows any viral infection. It most commonly follows Epstein-Barr virus infection and Coxsackie virus infection (Bornholm disease or epidemic myalgia).

2. The age distribution of patients shows two peaks at 25-29 years and 40-44 years. Both sexes are equally affected.

3. Symptoms of PVFS are many and varied. Any system of the body may be involved. Fatigue is the most common complaint, but fatigue on its own is insufficient to make the diagnosis.

4. Diagnosis of PVFS should be made by a doctor. A strict definition of PVFS should be used. If one considers only fatigue, the patient is most likely to have a psychiatric disorder.

5. Routine investigations should be performed on all patients. In individual patients, other investigations may be indicated after a detailed history and clinical examination has been performed.

6. Patients may take years to recover and should plan for gradual recovery rather than instant cure. Support from

relatives and friends on this basis is much more constructive.

7. The solution to patients' problems is first to recognise their situation. Patients are in many vicious circles which some refuse to recognise. A recognition of these circles is the key to developing a plan for better recovery.

8. Better recovery is only slow and gradual. A change of lifestyle is critical. It is not sufficient to read this book. Patients need to change their behaviour.

CHAPTER FIVE
FIRST STEP: MIND OUT

There is the story of Wee Ted who entered the tree-felling competition at the Lumberjack World Championships. Ahead of him were tall, massive lumberjacks who were able to cut a tree down in 20 seconds. When Wee Ted's turn came, there was mocking laughter everywhere. Amazingly, he cut his tree down in 10 seconds. The audience was aghast, and one lumberjack said:

"Where did you learn to fell trees like that?"

"The Sahara," Wee Ted replied.

"But there are no trees in the Sahara," quipped another lumberjack.

"Not any more," replied Wee Ted.

Patients with PVFS have to be like Wee Ted and have faith in themselves, even when the available evidence seems to be against them. They will be surrounded by apparently more able and knowledgeable people. Yet, the truth is what matters. If they know what their problems are and what has caused them, they must believe in themselves. **This is more difficult, but more sensible than taking advice from well-wishers who have no understanding of the problem.** One must remember that most people have little experience of delayed recovery after a viral illness. The mind is the part of the person that is responsible for thoughts, feeling and intentions. The mind is a major factor in determining a patient's recovery from PVFS. **"Mind out" means "to be careful" or "pay attention" and accurately describes what is required of PVFS patients.**

EMOTIONS

There is the age-old conundrum: what came first, the chicken or the egg? The relationship of emotion and immunity is complex. Patients' emotional state may influence the function of their immune system. Immunological abnormalities such as reduced levels of IgA immunoglobulins and increased T (helper) cells have been found in individuals under stress. **It is possible that patients' emotional state may predispose them to a viral infection, and to delayed recovery from that infection.**

Alternatively, it may be argued that before the illness, patients were well and that it is the illness itself which has produced the emotional abnormalities. Further, the other social and work consequences of the illness may also produce such effects, even if the initial illness does not. Suffice to say, in PVFS patients, there is usually a history of a viral infection and abnormal emotions. Like the chicken and the egg analogy, **the PVFS patient has to cope with the aftermath of a viral infection and emotions; what came first is academic.** Nevertheless, most PVFS patients do not have a history of great emotional disturbances. In studies in which about 75% of hospital

PVFS patients have a psychiatric disorder, the patients have usually been ill for years; in studies of recently-ill PVFS patients, the presence of a psychiatric disorder is considerably less and most are emotionally well (Shanks MF and Ho-Yen DO, British Journal of Psychiatry 1995; 166: 798-801). **Our study also argued against any simple theory of psychological causation or maintenance of PVFS.** Nevertheless, patients find themselves with many emotional problems:

	Problem	Frequency
1.	Fatigue	Always
2.	Depression	Common
3.	Anxiety	Common
4.	Paranoia	Rare
5.	Suicide	Very rare

FATIGUE

The most common complaints of PVFS patients are fatigue (asthenia) or tiredness. Associated complaints are malaise and weakness (lassitude). Malaise is a general feeling of ill-health. Weakness is the patient's perception that the muscles have reduced strength. **Fatigue is a state of tiredness in which the patient lacks energy and is unable to do much.** Obviously, fatigue and weakness blend into each other, and sometimes they cannot be separated.

Of patients' complaints, fatigue and weakness are the most frequent and complex. This is not surprising as these symptoms are a description of ill people. More than half the admissions to a general hospital will also have these complaints. However, for many doctors these symptoms may also suggest psychiatric illness, especially if the results of laboratory tests are negative. **Thus, many PVFS patients may at some stage be referred to a psychiatrist.**

As stated previously (Chapter Four), PVFS patients require more than fatigue before the diagnosis can be made. Indeed, a great mistake of the uninformed is that they tend to assume that PVFS patients have only fatigue. With strict diagnostic criteria, in patients with fatigue for a long time, only 4% have PVFS (Figure 7); the majority of patients who complain of only fatigue will have a psychiatric disorder. **If these facts were more widely known, many mistakes by the public and media would be avoided.**

PSYCHIATRIC DISORDERS

Many PVFS patients could develop some of the complaints of psychiatric disorders. The nature of PVFS, the loss of good health, the length of the illness and the lack of quick treatments may all combine to have adverse effects on patients. **Patients should be aware that there are several time bombs: depression, anxiety, paranoia and suicide.** Fortunately, most patients do not develop full-blown psychiatric disorders.

1. Depression
Depression or unhappiness is a common human emotion. It is a normal, healthy reaction to some of life's problems. It is only a medical problem when it is uncontrollable or if there is no obvious cause for the

depression. **Thus, for PVFS patients, it is not abnormal to be occasionally depressed about tiredness and easy fatigue, indeed it is normal and even necessary.** But, if this depression occurs all the time, then, the behaviour is abnormal. The situation is further complicated by the fact that depression itself can cause tiredness and fatigue.

2. Anxiety

Anxiety is a feeling of unease, apprehension, uncertainty and fear. With anxiety, unlike ordinary fear, the unease is out of proportion to the reason for the fear. Thus, PVFS patients may be anxious about going shopping or being in large crowds. Indeed, in such situations many have panic attacks. **Panic attacks are sudden, short-lived anxiety attacks.** Although this may be difficult to understand, I believe that in PVFS, panic attacks are a reflection of the increased concentration required for such activities, and the patients' realisation that they may not be able to cope. **Such patients are often able to easily cope with these situations when they start to recover.**

3. Paranoia

Paranoia is the development of feelings of suspicion and wariness of those around. There is a tendency to blame others and gradually delusions develop, with feelings of self-importance and entitlement. PVFS patients find it difficult to understand how those around can have only a very limited interest in their predicament. Relatives and friends are quickly bored, and they try to distance themselves from the patient. Patients may begin to feel that there is no one that they can talk to about their illness. **Patients then become suspicious of those around,**

imagining that others are speaking about them. There is increased wariness in the relationship from both parties and gradual deterioration of friendships.

4. Suicide
Fortunately for most patients, this is only a fleeting thought. Patients' lives can become so disrupted and disturbed that there may be little attraction in life. Each day, patients get up hoping to be cured. When this does not happen, they can feel abandoned and without hope. Their friends and relatives do not appreciate their frustration. Rapidly, patients can become isolated and lonely. **The world has little attraction. In this situation, contemplation of suicide is not surprising and can even appear to be a logical solution to many problems.** Fortunately, the vast majority of patients reject suicide. This is probably because PVFS patients usually have a great zest for life, and suicidal feelings can quickly pass.

5. Conclusion
Psychological problems, therefore can be an inherent part of PVFS. **However, psychological disorders are definitely *not* the cause of PVFS.** The symptoms and the length of illness may suggest to doctors that the patient has a psychiatric disorder, and indeed in some patients viral infections may precipitate anxiety and depression (Shanks MF and Ho-Yen DO, British Journal of Psychiatry, 1995; 166: 798-801). As the illness continues, the patient can develop more symptoms which can have the effect of making psychological problems worse. It is a vicious circle from which patients need to escape. **The first step involves patients believing in themselves and minding out.**

ASSOCIATED DISORDERS

1. Psychiatric Disorders

Psychiatric disorders are associated with PVFS. This means that in PVFS patients, a small number may develop a psychiatric disorder. Similarly, in patients with a psychiatric disorder a small number may develop PVFS. **Psychiatric disorders are not the cause of PVFS.** There are several other conditions which are associated with PVFS. The relationships between these syndromes and PVFS are depicted in Figure 9.

2. Primary Fibromyalgia Syndrome

This is an illness in which there are very tender areas in characteristic sites in a patient's body. The illness is usually chronic and there is evidence that many patients have an abnormal sleeping pattern (Ho-Yen DO, Physician 1990: 581-583). Medical practitioners must differentiate these two illnesses. **It is important to distinguish this condition from PVFS as the management is different.**

3. Tension Headaches

These are believed to be a result of stress on an individual. In individuals with tension headaches, fatigue is usually a minor complaint, and these patients can be completely well in the absence of stress. PVFS patients may develop such headaches and they may last weeks, and the headaches can be very resistant to treatment. **However, in PVFS the headaches are principally a result of over-activity, although stress may be an influential factor.** Headaches in PVFS are managed symptomatically and with bed rest.

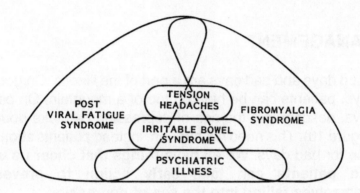

Figure 9 Important conditions associated with PVFS
Patients with fibromyalgia syndrome, tension headaches, irritable
bowel syndrome or psychiatric disorders may develop PVFS. This is
probably because infections occur in any group of patients. Similarly,
PVFS patients may go on to develop these associated conditions.

65

4. Irritable Bowel Syndrome

The situation here is quite different. **A large number of PVFS patients have abdominal complaints, especially alternating diarrhoea and constipation.** In addition, abdominal pain, "fullness" or "bloating" after a meal are common. In many patients the muscles in the gastrointestinal tract are probably affected.

MANAGEMENT

Good days and bad days are a part of the illness. On good days, patients can be high on top of a mountain. On bad days, descent into the sea of depression can take hours (Figure 10). This need not happen, instead patients should plan for bad days. **We all have things that cheer us up and patients can take early action to prevent themselves falling into the sea of depression.**

These actions seem so trivial that they are often not even considered by the patient. **Yet, this approach works. The essence is to recognise that *early* action is required.** Patients should put aside a variety of obstacles to depression (Figure 10). These may be: favourite videos (especially cartoons); jokes that have been particularly funny; pets whose antics make you laugh; or, food that makes you happy, even if it is a special chocolate. I recommend "It's good to laugh" by Graham Kennedy and Lynda Poole from the Persistent Virus Disease Research Foundation. Remember that prevention is better than a cure.

Recordings on a tape recorder or video of favourite programmes on radio or television are particularly useful. However, similar enjoyment may be obtained from looking

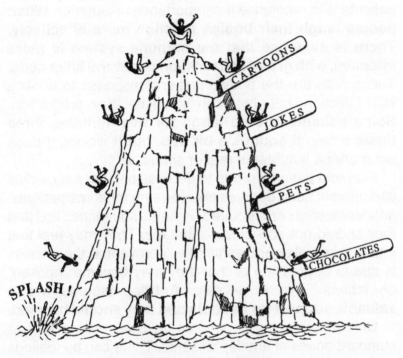

HIGH

CARTOONS

JOKES

PETS

CHOCOLATES

SPLASH!

SEA OF DEPRESSION

Figure 10   Sea of depression
Many patients tumble down from a high at the top of a mountain into
the sea of depression. This need not happen. Instead, a choice of
cartoons, jokes, pets and even food (such as chocolate) can be
effective obstacles to clinical depression.

at travel brochures, or reading a passage in a book about an odd place or situation. **Patients who are prone to becoming depressed should collect things that make them laugh.** An important aspect of managing PVFS patients is to recognise the importance of laughter. **When people laugh their bodies function more effectively. There is evidence that the immune system is more effective, with greater circulation of natural killer cells.** These cells are the body's first line response to dealing with infection. Laughter can stimulate their production. **Some patients should laugh for five minutes, three times a day. It sounds a bit odd, but it works.** It does not matter if laughter is real or simulated.

For most patients prone to depression, these remedies can prevent deep depression. However for some patients, antidepressants are required. Patients sometimes feel that they should not accept such therapy. They may feel that if they take antidepressants, it will prove that their illness is due to depression or that they may become "hooked" on tablets. This is unlikely. **Antidepressants are a valuable support for patients and they should be used.**

Unfortunately, many patients have adverse effects to standard doses of antidepressants. There can be feelings of "heaviness", "drowsiness" or "being a zombie." Yet, smaller doses of these same medicines can produce dramatic benefits as many patients have a great sensitivity to these drugs, **antidepressants should be given at minimal dosages.** Also, they should not be given long term and 3-6 month courses are best.

SUMMARY

1. PVFS patients have to believe in themselves. They must "mind out" and care for themselves.

2. A patient's emotional state may predispose to viral infections and delayed recovery.

3. Fatigue (asthenia) or tiredness are common complaints of patients with psychiatric disorders. PVFS patients are easily distinguished from psychiatric patients by the case definition of PVFS.

4. Psychiatric disorders (depression, anxiety, paranoia, suicide) are often a result of the illness. PVFS is not caused by psychiatric disorders.

5. A number of conditions are associated with PVFS: psychiatric disorders, primary fibromyalgia syndrome, tension headaches and irritable bowel syndrome.

6. Patients should adopt strategies to prevent depression. They should collect things that make them laugh, and remember that early treatment is critical in avoiding a more serious illness.

7. Antidepressants may be of great value to some patients. As patients are sensitive to these drugs, they should be given in low dosage.

CHAPTER SIX

SECOND STEP: ACQUIRE KNOWLEDGE

Brian was a man who did not like to spend money. He was reknown for taking lemonade bottles back to the shop, and using candles instead of electric lights at night. Yet, Brian was a very handsome man, and beautiful women were immediately attracted to him. Unfortunately, after a short time, these women could not cope with his stinginess.

One day he was waiting for a bus. When the bus finally arrived, he asked the conductor how much it was to the bus terminal.

"Fifty pence" said the conductor.

This was too much for Brian, so he decided to run behind the bus for the next two stops, and then asked:

"How much is it to the bus terminal now?" "Still fifty pence" replied the conductor.

Brian ran a further five stops – just to make sure that it would be cheaper and asked:

"How much is it now?"

"Eighty pence" said the conductor, "You're running in the wrong direction."

Many patients, even with the very best intentions, are

running in the wrong direction. Most PVFS patients have not had a simple explanation of what they have to do. Many are faced with too complicated advice; alternatively, there is the "there is nothing to be done" advice or "the disease will burn itself out". **These are all wrong.**

PVFS patients need to acquire knowledge of their illness to recover. This is because their illness is individual and only the patient can truly understand the many individual facets of the illness. However, acquisition of knowledge is not easy. Five types of knowledge, with their degree of difficulty are:

Knowledge	Difficulty
1. Illness (general)	Low
2. Illness (detailed)	Medium
3. Self	High
4. Individual PVFS effects	High
5. Daily diary	Very High

It is readily apparent that apart from general knowledge of the illness, none of these tasks are easy. Indeed, most tasks are of a high or very high degree of difficulty. If a patient is able to acquire the knowledge, the next step is to apply the knowledge. **When knowledge is applied to the illness, patients can develop control of the illness.** With this control, there is a greater confidence and the realisation that recovery is possible. From this realisation, it is a short step to knowing that recovery will soon come.

GENERAL KNOWLEDGE

General knowledge of the illness is relatively easy to acquire. For many, this can be simply reading a newspaper or magazine article about the illness. Many patients are happy to just try to establish that the illness exists. **At this stage, they may feel that if they find any more information, they may be accused of wanting to be ill.** Sadly, the effects of the illness make people defensive.

Patients' perceptions of the illness can be illogical. Many times patients have admitted to me that they did not like the diagnosis of PVFS and would rather if I said that they had a cancer. **This attitude is totally different to the general public's belief that PVFS patients would choose the diagnosis of PVFS rather than be well.** This is yet another example of the divide between reality and its perception. Patients need to acquire professional status rather than continuing to be amateurs. They need to have detailed knowledge rather than what is generally available. **The problem is major; patients need to become serious.**

DETAILED KNOWLEDGE

Detailed knowledge of the illness is not easily acquired and involves a medium degree of difficulty. Patients will have to try and understand all of their symptoms. They will need to read a book about their illness. With this greater knowledge, patients will be able to see their illness as a whole. **Sadly many patients see their illness as only bad news** (Figure 11). It requires a great effort to even start to look for information with this attitude in mind.

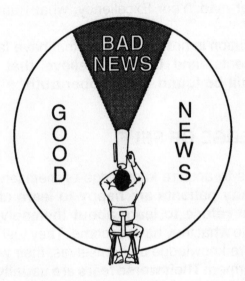

PATIENT'S LIFE

Figure 11 Patient's life

Many patients can only see the bad news in their life. Illness has created a limited vision. Part of recovery depends on patients being able to see their whole illness. Many will then recognise that there is more good news than bad news.

Pope has said:

"A little learning is a dangerous thing; Drink deep, or taste not the Pierian spring". I once mentioned this quotation to a patient who replied by quoting from the Bible:

"Too much learning doth make thee mad" (Acts 26:24).

It is perhaps instructive to remember that the above statement was made by someone attacking Paul, and that Paul had replied:

"I am not mad, Your Excellency, what I am saying is sober truth".

This situation is not unlike those that have faced many PVFS patients, and **I firmly believe that the best answers will be found in the sober truth.**

KNOWLEDGE OF SELF

For patients to acquire knowledge of themselves is very difficult. **Many patients are happy to learn about their illness, but refuse to learn about themselves.** Often, patients hate what they have become. They feel that if they acquire more knowledge of themselves, their worse fears will be confirmed. **Their worse fears are usually that they would not be able to be active again.**

Patients remember their past life and cannot bear to look at their present position. **They are essentially mourning the death of their past existence.** As with all mourning, their ability to face the facts is limited. They refuse to accept that their past existence is over. **Yet, for recovery, patients need to understand what is happening and recognise their mourning.**

Fortunately, for most patients their past existence is not as important as they perceive it. With time and honesty, it will be recognised that they often lived on adrenaline. As all drugs, it can be addictive. Yet, it is possible to be happy and content without adrenaline. **Recovery can depend on patients being able to recognise that in the past they depended on activity and adrenaline for a "high".** One patient said that he was happy only when car racing. Then, he felt no pain, nor tiredness. He often won. Usually this was followed by two weeks in bed – the after effects of the adrenaline. The same adrenaline which allowed him to have no pain nor tiredness.

INDIVIDUAL EFFECTS

When sufferers talk among themselves, they realise that they have great similarities as well as great differences in their illnesses. **It is very unusual to find two patients with exactly the same complaints.** This does not mean that different patients have different illnesses. Instead, it should be realised that a patient's complaints are individual (Figure 12). The illness has such widespread effects on the body that complaints are many and varied.

I am often amazed at the paradox of patients' perception of their past and current lives. In the past, they were productive, active and triumphed in their individuality. **Currently, as they are not productive or active, they want to be exactly the same as other sufferers.** The only way that they are the same as before is in their individuality, but they want to reject this only similarity with the past. It is a symptom of the lack of confidence that comes with illness. Somehow it is no longer possible to wear the scarlet tie or scarf.

PATIENT GROUP

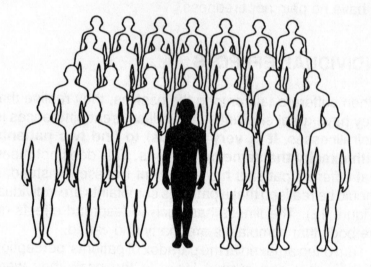

Figure 12
In a large group of PVFS patients, each patient's complaints will be slightly different. For each patient, the illness will have individual effects. This is why it is important for patients to acquire personal knowledge of their illness.

DAILY DIARY

Most patients were previously well-organised individuals who prided themselves on their abilities to solve problems. Sadly, when memory and/or concentration are affected, a once efficient individual may behave like a headless chicken. When people succeed in life, they often have an edge. It may be in ability, organisation or luck. Usually success is a reflection of accentuating one's strengths and minimising the effects of one's weaknesses. **It therefore makes sense to compensate for poor memory by keeping a daily diary.**

A daily diary is very hard to keep and this is the most difficult task. Many patients and their relatives regard a daily diary as "patients wallowing in their illness." I cannot accept this argument. Recovery depends on knowledge; and without a diary, how do you know if you are running in the right direction? Patients often reply that they know that they are getting worse. **If patients are getting worse, they are obviously running in the wrong direction.**

There are several difficulties in keeping a daily diary:

	Problem	Difficulty
1.	Desire	High
2.	Format	Low
3.	Regularity	Medium
4.	Content	Low
5.	Precision	Medium
6.	Scoring system	High
7.	Learning	High

For an ill individual, the above may appear formidable. Yet, overall it is not a difficult task – with help. **I have not found a patient who is unable to keep a good diary.** Indeed, many children can be taught to produce excellent diaries. However, patients must first want to help themselves.

1. Desire

Many patients initially accept the need for a diary, but after a week they cannot be bothered. **I feel that the diary is so important that I would refuse to see a patient who did not keep a diary.** Apart from the reasons given above, I can tell how a patient has been over six weeks in 5 minutes if the patient has a diary. If there is no diary, the same information takes 45-60 minutes to acquire. The desire to keep a diary is of high difficulty because patients have no energy to keep a diary, and they feel that their lives are so boring that there is no help in a diary. Patients often say "every day is exactly the same," "all I do is rest" or "I have no energy to do anything." Yet, some patients get better and others do not. **In patients who are getting worse, there are usually several things that they are doing wrong.** The fastest way for me to find out what they are doing wrong is to examine a daily diary.

The daily diary that I like takes 3 minutes per day to keep. This is not a large amount of time. I believe that if patients cannot give 3 minutes per day for their diary, it is not surprising that they are not getting better. **The diary must also be written by the patient.** I am often told "my wife/husband will do the diary" or "my mother/father is good at writing." **However, I always insist on the patient doing the diary.** Even young children can be taught to keep a useful diary. It is also a measure of the patient's commitment to getting better.

2. Format

The format of the diary is depicted in Figures 13 and 14. **A school exercise book is best as you can write on both sides of the paper.** It is better than photocopying the format, although photocopying reduces some work, it is not as easy to refer to or use. **Two pages should be used for each week: one page for scores (Figure 13) and the next page for the patient's activities (Figure 14).** The scoring system is explained later in this chapter. Sometimes patients feel that they want to write more. This is good but it is important that this diary be on one page, and often patients who like to write more will keep two diaries. In another diary, they may go into greater detail and even record more private matters. **My agreement with patients is simply that they keep a daily diary.** It is of tremendous importance and takes only 3 minutes per day.

3. Regularity

Initially, patients may write 2-3 pages in their diary when they are feeling well; and if they have a relapse there will be blank pages, they will reply with indignation:

"I did nothing, so I wrote nothing!" This is not good enough. **I only require two lines each day, but I need these two lines every day of the year.** If the daily diary is not kept, it is of limited use.

The format of my diary is designed to be simple. It can be done even though patients are very ill. Many patients remark at how simple the diary appears. Yet, this is usually when patients have a lot to say. The diary can be very difficult for an individual who is in relapse. **However, I have only rarely encountered a patient who is unable to keep a daily diary despite the seriousness**

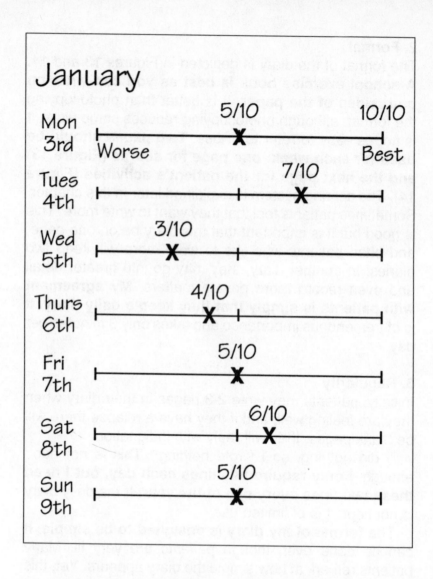

Figure 13 Left-hand page of the diary
One page is used for each week. On the left-hand page of the exercise book, daily scores are kept of how the patient feels on a scale of 1–10.

Mon   Sleep 12hr. Hospital. Travel (2hrs)
         Sleep afternoon (3hrs) TV (1hr) Bad day.

Tues Sleep 14hrs. Short walk (1/2hr) Visitors x2
         Telephone x3. TV (3hrs) Good day.

Wed Sleep 8hrs Bad night. Very tired
         Back to bed (6hrs) TV (2hrs) Terrible.

Thurs Sleep 8hrs. Disturbed night. Read (1hr)
         Unwind (x2) TV (2hrs) Boredom (X2) Better.

Fri   Sleep 12hrs. Read (2hrs) Unwind (x2)
         Telephone (x2) Boredom (x3) Boring day.

Sat   Sleep 14hrs. Argument with mother (11/2hrs)
         Shopping (2hrs) Telephone (x2) Fair day.

Sun   Sleep 10hrs. Church (2hrs) Visitors x2
         Unwind (x1) TV (3hrs) Average day.

Figure 14 Right-hand page of the diary
One page is used for each week. On the right-hand page, two lines
describe the patient's day. Do not write in sentences. Record hours
of sleep and relaxation, activities, visitors, telephone calls, problems
and how you feel.

81

of the relapse. A daily diary is the cornerstone for better recovery.

4. Content

Although this is of low difficulty, many patients find this is a problem. A major consideration is that many patients remember how active they were, and feel that in comparison there is nothing to write. Although such an approach is logical, it does not deal with the problem. **The problem is simply that without detailed daily information, a patient's chance of recovery is greatly diminished.**

It is easier if patients have a systematic approach to the content of a diary. Firstly, there is no need to write in sentences. It is only 2-3 lines and therefore it needs to contain as much information as possible. State the important facts first: hours of sleep, hours of relaxation and if you are having a period (menstruation). Next, record how you have spent your time in hours of television, radio, reading newspapers or books; and record your number of visitors and telephone calls. Lastly, say how you feel (happy, unhappy, good, bad etc). **Do not become discouraged about your diary.** With time, you will develop an understanding of what should be in the diary. Like many skills in life, a diary takes time and effort. The reward is better recovery from PVFS.

5. Precision

Many diaries start off being emotional rather than precise. Frequent comments are: "This is hell on earth," "I am about to die," "I've never experienced such torture," "When will I find peace?" and "The pain is unbearable". However, to be of value, a diary needs to be precise. So, more useful comments would be: "I can't get out of bed," "I can only walk 100 yards," "I had diarrhoea ten times today," or "My headache lasted 12 hours."

A precise diary allows comparison over time. One or two years later, patients may be able to go back and see how they were. I am always surprised that patients are quite happy to say to me:

"I have not been well for years and it is getting worse each year."

Yet, when I asked them when it started, there is usually a blank stare. When I ask how it has got worse over each six-month period, there is a look of astonishment that I might require such information. **Without such information it is impossible to predict the future progress of the illness.**

6. Scoring system

Patients need to have an overall impression of how they are. This takes time. The first difficulty is that patients feel differently at different times of the day. Some are worse in the morning; others are worse at night. Some patients often feel that they should score themselves in the morning, afternoon, evening and at night. This is too complicated. **Patients should learn to develop an overall average score for the day.** This is the easiest and most useful approach.

The scoring system is:

Score Effects
1. Severe symptoms at rest. In bed all day.
2. Moderate to severe symptoms at rest. Feels unable to work. Concentration and activity severely affected.

3. Moderate symptoms at rest. Feels unable to work full-time. Activities severely affected.
4. Mild symptoms at rest. Feels just able to work full-time but not in a physical or stressful job. Frequent rest/relaxation needed.
5. Very mild symptoms at rest. Moderate to severe symptoms with exercise or activity. Feels able to work full-time, but not in a physical or stressful job. Social life restricted.
6. Very mild or no symptoms at rest. Moderate symptoms with exercise. Feels able to work full-time, but not in a physical job. Social life affected.
7. Very mild or no symptoms at rest. Mild symptoms, with exercise. Feels able to work full-time but not in a physical job. Some social life.
8. No symptoms at rest. Very mild or no symptoms with some exercise. Feels able to work full-time in a reasonably active job. Some social life.
9. No symptoms at rest. Few symptoms with exercise. Feels able to work full-time in a reasonably active job. More social life.
10. Patient well.

The scoring system is rated as being of high difficulty. This is because there are several problems which patients have:

a) **Feel before you do:** Scores are what you feel or think that you can do. It is not about what you can do. Many patients do not want to score a number until they can do it; as these patients tend to overdo things, they may never reach higher than 5. You must feel that you might be able to do something for

84

several weeks before you try it.

b) **Have before you spend:** The left-hand side of the diary is your income and the right-hand side is how you spend it. You must have high scores before you do more. Most patients want to spend it first (on credit) and promise themselves that they will pay it back after the event. This is wrong. There is no spending on credit as you are already bankrupt. You must have high scores **before** you go to the event. If you do not have a high score, you cannot go. This discipline is critical for recovery.

c) **Wanting to be precise:** using decimal places (5.1 or 4.35). Patients should stick to whole numbers, occasionally halves or quarters are acceptable.

d) **Changes in a week:** it is useful to look at a week and see one day that was better or worse than the rest. Thus, to see seven 5's is not as useful as five 5's, one 4 and one 6. Overall for the week the score is the same. Do not be afraid of using a range of numbers.

e) **Wanting to change past scores:** patients often say "last year this time I scored 5, but it was not really a 5, it was a 3; I am now a 5." The score that is correct is the score that you **feel** now. A year from now, if you feel better you should score yourself higher, rather than go back to the diary and change the previous year's scores.

f) **Fear of being too optimistic:** there is an irrational

fear of scoring higher scores. It is not unlike the teacher who cannot give students full marks. The scoring system has guidelines but patients should score themselves relative to the previous days/weeks.

CONTROLLING SCORES

Many patients feel that they have no control of scores. It is as though they were counting cars passing along a street and had no control of the cars. My approach is to let them feel that they control the traffic lights for the street. They can let no cars pass or choose the rate at which cars pass. **It is a big step when the diary is not just a record but a result of a patient's ability to control his/her behaviour during the day.**

It takes time to develop the skills required to control diary scores. Over many years, patients have particularly benefitted from:

a) **The future.** The discipline of remaining within your energy levels is not easy. But, what is the reason for such discipline? The reason is so that you get better faster. Thus it is important to remind yourself: "I must be disciplined. My future depends on it. What I do today affects what I will be two months from now." The philosophy must be to sacrifice today for tomorrow.

b) **Contracts.** Making a contract with yourself can be a tremendous boost in controlling diary scores. Say, for example, that you would not go on the computer (or visit your mother) unless you score half a point above your average of the previous month. Do not set too difficult conditions, but they must not be too easy either! If you can start to enjoy these contracts, life can become easier. Also, it may not be any more restrictive than saying you will only have a barbecue on a sunny day.

c) **Early stops.** The ability to stop before you run out of energy is very hard for most patients. They stay at the party too long or must watch the last half hour of the video. The fact that their minds are totally out of it, unable to concentrate or take part is not considered. Worse, the after-effects may influence scores for the next week. It is madness. It is better to adopt an "early stop" approach. As soon as the battery dims, turn the torch off and put the battery in the recharger. As soon as you become tired, go to bed.

d) **Crisis management.** Managing a bad day is crisis management. On bad days, it is important to make yourself laugh several times. Also you must not make bad days worse: it is not worth attempting a trip, difficult meeting or visit on a bad day. If you can remain within your energy limits and laugh a few times, a bad day (the crisis) will be efficiently managed.

e) **"Blow outs".** In any system, there must be some time for a "blow out". Obviously it is best that these are planned so it is better if you invite the guests to dinner rather than they turn up uninvited. It is not bad to have a small blow out once a week, and perhaps a bigger indulgence once a month. It is also a nice feeling to plan a small blow out, but not do it. Instead, save it for another time when you might need it more.

LEARNING

Patients usually do the diary because I ask them. **It is useful to me, but it should be more useful to the patient.** When the diary scores are bad, patients should do less. Thus the diary scores influence their behaviour in subsequent days. **Learning from the diary is the most difficult lesson.** Patients are often content to keep very detailed diaries, but not to let the diary influence their behaviour.

The diary is a key to answering many questions. Not all female patients feel worse during menstruation, but some do – the diary can provide the answer. One patient used the diary to realise that visiting her father made her worse. Another, detected a food allergy. **Patients need to use the diary to learn.**

Keeping such records can be demanding but they are necessary. A detailed diary shows an outsider that you are concerned about your illness and you are trying to be objective. But more important, a diary can be a tremendous boost when you are going through a difficult time. It is reassuring to be able to know how you compare to 1, 3 or 5 years ago. **Most patients over this period will have stayed the same, although comparisons over shorter periods (weeks or months) may show deterioration.** The problems can also change with time and here a diary can be instructive. One patient was almost suicidal about her health and, from her diary, indicated that in a 3-year period she had had ten different complaints. When it was pointed out that she had overcome 9 problems, her retort was a predictable "There were 9 too many!" **Being objective about one's illness is difficult. It takes time, and one does not know if it is worth it.** But what is the alternative? To sit around waiting for a miracle?

Detailed recording of symptoms is the second step to better recovery from viral infections. Specific knowledge about oneself will allow a change of attitude and lifestyle. **Great strength can come from the realisation that self-help is possible and that many solutions to problems are within one's capabilities.** Whereas recovery may take years, life can be better now. It just needs a positive start.

SUMMARY

1. Patients often feel that if they acquire too much information about their illness, they may be accused of wanting to be ill.

2. Patients require to have detailed knowledge of their illness. They need to learn that their illness is not only bad news, and the best answers will be found in the sober truth.

3. Patients often have fears of knowing themselves. Many mourn their past existence and believe that they have no worth when they are ill.

4. PVFS patients are individual and it is unusual to find two patients with the same complaints. Before illness, patients prided themselves on their individuality; with

illness, patients want to be like everyone else. It is a reflection of a loss of confidence.

5. A daily diary allows patients to know if they are making progress. It is difficult to keep a daily diary, but first patients must want to record detailed information. The diary takes 3 minutes/day, and is not a long time for patients to devote to getting better.

6. Ideally, an exercise book should be used with two pages for each week. The diary should be kept daily. It should record the activities in the day, and a scoring system should be used. Scores reflect what you feel and not what you can do. Also, you must have high scores before you do more.

7. There are several ways of controlling scores, and patients must put these into practice.

8. The most important result of a daily diary is when a patient learns from the diary. The diary is not mainly for the doctor, but for the patient.

CHAPTER SEVEN

THIRD STEP:
LOSING ENERGY: EXERCISE, STRESS AND RELATIONSHIPS

In 1831, George Osbaldeston bet 1000 guineas that he could travel by horse faster than Stephenson's new Rocket locomotive. At the time, the Rocket travelled at the record speed of 24 miles per hour, and no one could see how Osbaldeston could win. Worse, the race was over 200 miles and Osbaldeston was handicapped. Forty-four years old, five foot tall with a badly crippled leg, he hardly looked capable of lasting the course. Amazingly, allowing for stops and riding 28 horses, he averaged 26 miles per hour and easily won his bet. At the end of the race, he announced that he was so hungry that he "could eat an old woman". Such feats of endurance have always had an attraction, and indeed, have a special section in the Guinness Book of Records.

Understanding energy is the most difficult step to better recovery. Patients usually regard energy as something to use, and cannot think of gaining or losing energy. Because of this problem, over many years I have developed a four-part strategy for teaching patients to understand energy:

1. Think of energy as money
2. Stop losing energy
3. Try gaining energy
4. Try making energy last.

The first two parts will be dealt with in this chapter, but separate chapters will be devoted to gaining energy (Chapter 8) and making energy last (Chapter 9).

ENERGY AS MONEY

The first part of the strategy is to think of energy as money. To get better, patients need to recognise that they cannot use more energy (or money) than they have. If they do, as with money, they will get worse (or go further into debt). Indeed, as patients are ill, they have a massive overdraft at the bank, so they need to save some money (or energy) each day. The first part of the strategy is explained in Figures 15 to 18. **My approach has worked with many patients over decades.**

In time, patients have to develop the ability of looking at all their activities in terms of money. It is not just physical activities, but also mental activities which use up energy. There is only £100 to spend in the day. **I do not care how you spend this money, but I care if you spend more than your £100.** If you want to go for an early morning walk and spend £50, that is fine. But you must remember that you do not have that money (energy) to use later in the day. Thus, it is more sensible to wait until the evening to see how much money you have left over for the walk. **Like money, if you make a note of all you spend, you will be aware of how easy it is to lose money (energy).**

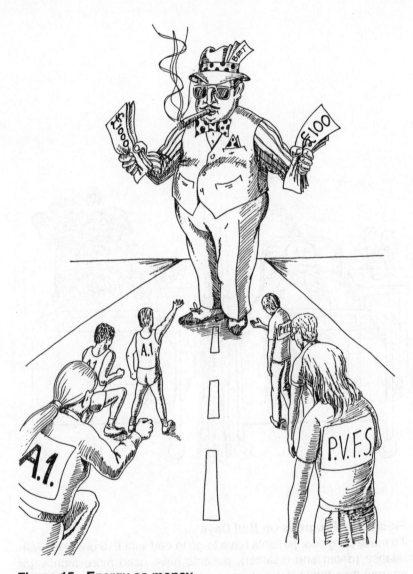

Figure 15 Energy as money
Patients should think that before the illness they had £1000 worth of energy for each day. With PVFS, they have £100 of energy for each day. Like someone losing their income, there has to be a severe cutback on activities.

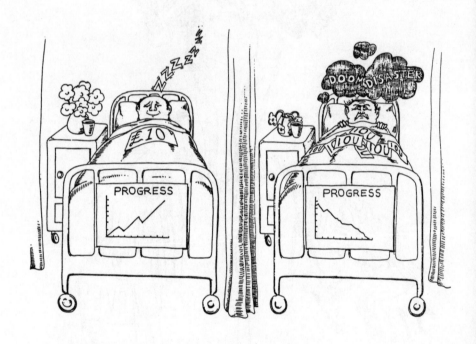

Figure 16 Progress on Bad Days
To make progress, patients have to go to bed with £10 unspent. With relapse (doom and disaster), patients have used more money (or energy) than they have and end up borrowing money.

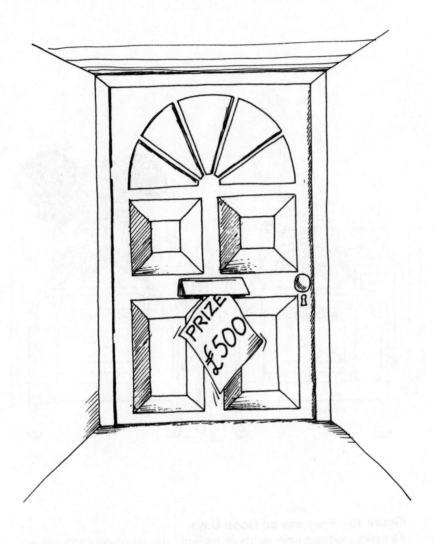

Figure 17   A Good Day
A good day is like receiving a £500 prize of energy. It is a great boost
and must be used wisely.

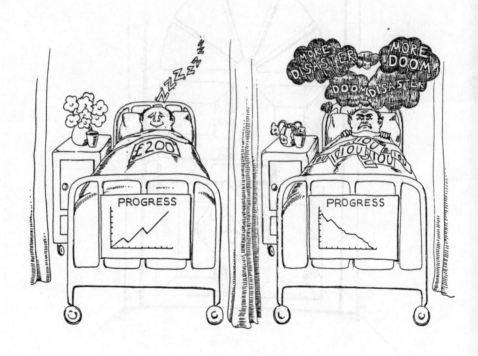

Figure 18   Progress on Good Days

To make progress on good days, patients should spend £300 and say that this amount is three times the bad days, and save £200. This repays the debt quicker and leaves something for tomorrow. Instead, patients usually try to catch up with activities, spend all of the £500 and end up borrowing more money. Greater doom and disaster are inevitable.

EXERCISE

Exercise itself is a complex subject, and as with religion, it means different things to different people. Many look upon exercise as extreme physical activity, and involves "going for the burn" or passing through a "pain barrier". I prefer the definition of exercise as "exertion of the body". It can be difficult for patients to recognise that they previously regarded only a five mile run as exercise, and I regard a 100 yard walk as exercise. The important factor is not the words used but the cost in energy. Thus, it does not matter if you went "shopping", but how much you spent; and there is a big difference between spending £1000 that you can afford and £10 which you cannot afford. **The important lesson for patients is that all exercise uses energy.**

There is the saying that "there are no free dinners". This means that even if something appears to be free, there is a hidden cost or commitment. It is a universal truth. Thus, for all patients, as with money, one must keep a record of outgoings and record all expenditure. **Then, the true cost of exercise and its value can be considered.** Recently, it has been recognised that many individuals can become addicted to exercise. There is addiction to the post-exercise high caused by endorphins released into the brain. These individuals take longer to recover from their training and their performances begin to suffer, often complicated by frequent infections. These individuals need to remember that **you are healthy only if you can recuperate adequately from training.** You do not get fit when you train, **you get fit when you recover from training.** Normally, muscles can take 20 hours to repair themselves. In PVFS patients, this time is greatly increased. **It is not surprising that patients cannot easily recover from training.**

THE ANSWER

What is the answer to excessive tiredness in PVFS? Two popular suggestions exist. The first is that the body is weak so it tires easily (because of exhaustion) as the patient is unfit. The second is that the body takes a long time to return to normal (because of delayed recovery), again due to the patient being unfit. Not surprisingly, many patients conclude that their tiredness is due to them being unfit; and if they became fit again, their tiredness would go away. In PVFS patients, there is no evidence to support this conclusion. **This reasoning applies to those with normal body function. The evidence in PVFS patients is that their body function is abnormal – they are ill.**

In normal muscles, the pain (or the burn) is due to the build up of lactic acid. Exercise gurus say of this: "There is absolutely nothing harmful or dangerous about it. It just slows you down until the oxygen supply is replenished, which is a matter of seconds." Using the technique of magnetic resonance imaging in PVFS patients, the muscles have been shown to form lactic acid more quickly and to take longer to get rid of it as compared to normal. This is probably a result of disordered metabolic regulation in the muscles – a result of the viral infection. **Thus, in PVFS patients, the reason for this tiredness is both exhaustion and delayed recovery.** Neither are caused by the patient being unfit, but rather, by the muscles behaving abnormally.

There is additional evidence of muscle abnormality.

Many PVFS patients have atypical muscle findings. The problems though are that results are non-specific and patients are at different stages of their illness. There is no doubt that the longer that you are ill, abnormalities are more likely to occur. At the moment, muscle abnormalities cannot be used for diagnosis. Also, the fact that not all patients demonstrate the same abnormalities is to be expected as several mechanisms may result in muscle dysfunction.

Although patients may accept that there are muscle abnormalities, many cannot believe that exercise is not the answer. As most individuals who develop PVFS were more athletic than normal, it is not surprising that they should look upon exercise as a solution to their problems. **In the past, they remember being fit – a time when they were able to exercise vigorously, and feel the better for it.** So, how can the question of exercise be answered for the individual patient?

This is where the diary is very useful. Looking at the tiredness (or other symptoms such as muscle pain) over a two month period, and attempting to relate this to physical exertion is an instructive lesson. In most patients, it is found that mild exercise, such as a 10 minute walk or a 5 minute swim, does not result in symptoms. Whereas, a hill walk for more than an hour, excessive physical activity, or lifting heavy weights can result in 2-7 days of tiredness. **With greater exercise other symptoms can also occur,** especially pain or burning in the muscles, diarrhoea, headaches, difficulty in seeing or hearing, and muscle twitches or tremors.

With the help of the diary, one can establish how much exercise can be tolerated and for how long. **The most important fact to realise is that there is considerable**

difference in what patients used to be able to do and what they can do now. For example, one patient enjoyed running 5 miles to work before his illness, but was only able to walk 10 yards without symptoms after his illness started. Many patients ignore their symptoms, and try to do exactly what they were capable of before their illness. The result is predictable, they feel unwell for the next 7-10 days. **Such forlorn attempts to emulate past achievements always take their toll.**

Patients have a difficulty in remembering that they are ill. If one's leg was in plaster, no one would contemplate running 5 miles. Like those around them, they have fallen into the trap of equating physical disability with illness. **The truth is that health is a reflection of what the body is capable of doing.** Well being is not what the body looks as though it can do, or what someone thinks that it should do.

The diary is particularly useful in showing relationships between symptoms and preceding events. It is best not to think of exercise as producing particular symptoms. **Whatever complaint the patient usually has is made worse by excessive exercise.** Exercise is an additional stress to the body and results in symptoms related to the activity, and worsening of existing complaints. Using the analogy of the battery, if the inside car lights are dim because of a poorly-charged battery, these lights become dimmer when the headlights are on full-beam. Generally, patients do not benefit from increasing exercise until they are 80% recovered. It is as though the body needs to recover in other ways before exercise can produce a benefit. **The important lesson is that exercise is a great way of losing energy.**

TYPE OF EXERCISE

The type of exercise is more important than the quantity and duration. **Some exercises use more money (energy) than others, so that an hour of squash is more exhausting than an hour of walking the dog.** Similarly, particular muscle groups can become overworked, so that half an hour chopping down a tree can have a more prolonged effect than the same time floating in the swimming pool. Team games in particular may require bursts of physical activity. **In general, the best type of exercise is one in which the exertion is constant, and capable of being controlled by the patient.** Thus, team games are not advisable, as it is usually not possible to go more slowly or stop. The best activity is one in which the patient controls the pace, however slow it may be.

Certain types of exercise, especially social ones tend to occur at the weekends. This can produce more noticeable effects. A patient with two exercise periods a week complained of excessive tiredness on Monday of each week. On further questioning, all of his activity was on Saturday and Sunday. When he changed his pattern to Saturday and Wednesday, his tiredness was dramatically reduced. Muscle groups that were previously well-developed (e.g. arms or legs; right-handedness or left-handedness) tend to be more severely affected. **Similarly, activities that an individual used to be good at are often more tiring than entirely new activities.** Human behaviour is such that when times are bad, there is a tendency to dig-in or fall-back (i.e. repeat current activity or go back to activities in the past). Both of these natural instincts may result in more tiredness than developing a new interest.

In 1985, I said that it can be helpful to look upon the body as a rechargeable battery. In the early stages of illness, it is a battery that cannot hold its charge for very long. Thus, exercise quickly results in exhaustion, and is followed by a prolonged period during which the body recharges itself. As the illness progresses, the body gradually improves and becomes a battery capable of holding its charge longer. Now, more exercise can be endured. **Exercise does not result in immediate tiredness, but often several days later, and recovery from tiredness is much faster.** Ideally, patients develop a feel for how much activity and the type of activity that can be tolerated. With the simile of the battery, they know how much charge is going to be used with each activity, and what the effects will be. There are times when they decide to exhaust themselves in the knowledge that recovery may take weeks. **These decisions are no worse than someone deciding to finish the punch at a party, and knowing that there will be a giant hangover for the next day.**

STRESS AND RELATIONSHIPS

There is a particular definition of stress that I like: **stress is a process in which the resources of the person are matched against the demands of the environment.** In my book, "Unwind" (Dodona Books, 1991), stress management techniques are carefully considered. Put simply, for chronically ill patients to cope with stress requires either reducing the demands of the environment or increasing their resources. **Resources can be increased by sleep and relaxation techniques**

(Chapter 8). Reducing the demands of the environment is much more difficult. Usually such demands are in three main areas: relationships, job and finances. Employment and finances are considered in Chapter 11.

Relationships, stress and energy needs can be considered as:

Relationships	Stress	Energy Needs
1. Friends	Low/Medium	Low/Medium
2. Relatives	Medium	Medium
3. Family	High	High
4. Partners	Very High	Very High

Obviously, a particularly annoying friend or relative can use more energy than a partner. Thus, the energy needs are approximate and are also a reflection of how I believe you should use your energy. **Thus, your partner should have most of your energy, followed by your family and lastly your friends.** Often, there is not enough energy for all, and patients have to choose their priorities.

One recent recognition is that energy is lost through mental activity. Although physical activity is the usual way money (energy) is spent, money is also lost through mental activity. **Thus, patients may stay in bed all day, but if they are worrying or anxious, energy is used up as if they were active.** Fortunately, mental activity uses energy more slowly than physical activity. However, this can be deceptive and many patients do not recognise that they are using energy. **The mental activities that use up much energy are: anger, hate, frustration, jealousy, depression and anxiety.** Sadly, these emotions are major factors in relationships.

FRIENDS

Friends can have difficulties coping with patients who are changed by the illness. It is not uncommon for a patient to say: **"I only started to get better when I lost all of my friends."** This is because friends remember patients as active, productive individuals. Often, these friends were very dependent on patients. As patients still look the same, their friends still have great expectations of patients. **Patients must be prepared to lose friends who are too demanding.**

Fortunately, there are some friendships in which the contributions of both individuals are about equal. These relationships are beneficial to the patients, and are the friendships that should be continued. There is a simple test. **One feels better after sharing some time with a good friend.** If you are angry, annoyed or frustrated after being with someone, you should question the relationship. With illness, patients have limited resources. Therefore, it makes sense to only do what is necessary. **If you can only afford to feed yourself, it is not possible for you to feed your friends.** But, one needs social contact, so it is better to choose friends who are happy to pay for their meal. Facing reality can be very difficult. It means that you may have to decide not to support others. **Patients should concentrate on those relationships that are mutually supportive.**

RELATIVES

Whereas we can choose our friends we cannot choose our relatives. For most patients, this is good news. **Friends**

often accept you for what you can do, but relatives accept you because you exist. The support of relatives for the vast majority of patients is overwhelming. **Help and assistance is usually freely given.** Without this support, many patients would have had great difficulties.

Sadly, this is not the whole story. There are many instances, especially with a daughter and an older parent, where the relationship is unhealthy. **Several ill patients feel compelled to support an older parent.** Patients can feel that it is their duty. There are usually great feelings of guilt. Often, the parent manipulates the patient and makes many unreasonable demands. The patient dreads visiting the parent and feels terrible after each visit. **My advice to these patients is simple: explain the situation to the parent and reduce the contact; do not feel guilty and do not be manipulated.**

Parents have a responsibility to care for their children; children do not have a responsibility to care for their parents. If children care for their parents, they should do so willingly and with love and not because of guilt. Many patients have said to me that they hated their parents; yet, they were prepared to care for the parent, thereby prolonging their illness. I have sadly concluded that if a parent has manipulated offspring for 20 – 30 years, they cannot stop when the offspring become ill. **Worse, when the offspring is ill, he/she is least able to withstand the demands of parents.**

FAMILY

In this section, I am considering the immediate family. **For patients, the family unit can determine whether they**

105

recover or not. The support of the family is invaluable, as the goodwill in the family is usually high. This goodwill is the key to being able to use the resources of the family.

With illness, the patient's role within the family has to change. No longer is it possible for the mother to do all of the housework, or the father to do the handyman jobs about the house. The whole family have to be recruited to help. Children, even as young as five years, can be taught to be helpful. **The great obstacle is accepting that the job will not be done properly.** However, it is still better for the patient if children only clean the kitchen 60% as well as the patient. **The patient needs to accept this help, and gently teach the children.** I have felt that with time and good teaching, the job can even be done better by the children. With all good teaching, the pupil should eventually perform better than the teacher.

PARTNERS

Partners (**or carers**) have a heavy, heavy burden. They see loved ones going through dramatic change: the active become inactive; the confident become afraid; the dependable become erratic; tears, anger and frustration become an everyday occurrence. For many it can be too much. **Many PVFS patients end up separated or divorced.** However, I am impressed at how many relationships survive and prosper. The relationships that do well have several common characteristics. These characteristics are probably necessary for all good relationships, however, with illness they can become vitally important.

Characteristics and Difficulties for a partner:

Characteristic	Difficulty
1. Mutual respect	Low
2. Consideration	Low
3. Understanding	Medium
4. Common objectives	Medium
5. Time together	High
6. Sexual activity	Very high

I have not used love, possibly because it is so hard to define. **If love is present many of the characteristics are also present, and the relationship will be good.** However, in many relationships in which there is said to be love, one finds one partner doing all the loving and the other consenting to be loved.

A good test of a relationship is the sexual activity, and in PVFS patients this has a very high degree of difficulty. **There are substantial differences between men and women.** With men, sexual activity is generally regarded as the main course of a three course meal; without the main course, there is no sustenance. With women, sexual activity is generally regarded as the dessert of a three course meal; sustenance is obtained with the main course, and the dessert is consumed if there is still hunger, time and inclination. **Couples need to rethink their sexual activity depending on which partner is affected.** This is a matter of great importance and cannot be left until a patient recovers.

A good sexual relationship is an aid to recovery, and a poor one is a large hindrance. Success depends on sexual activity when there is energy and the time is right. This usually means that sex is better in the morning or after lunch rather than at night. It should not be rushed, patients need time for arousal. **It is a mistake to think of only touching each other during sexual activity.** Often, there are good reasons for this, such as a patient being in a lot of pain. However, if there is love, a gentle touch can be a powerful analgesic, cuddles should also be part of a healthy relationship, and need not necessarily lead to the sexual act. Many women find greater enjoyment out of cuddles compared to the sexual act. **Muscle and joint pain can be obstacles to sexual activity.** Gentle massage of the affected partner is often a prelude to sex and can reduce pain. Couples will also need to experiment with various sexual positions. Side by side can be a useful position, and do not be afraid of using pillows to support tender areas such as the neck or lower back. **Couples should experiment and be open in their discussion of each experiment.**

If the patient is the man, the situation is slightly easier. Some patients find it difficult to maintain an erection, but matters are helped if the woman is first well-lubricated. Again, a useful position is with the woman on top. **Both partners will need to develop great patience.** When the patient is a woman, there may be a need to consider sex differently. Most women consider quality rather than quantity. Whereas, men would usually prefer to eat bread regularly rather than starve apart from feasts on good days. A solution is for the patient to masturbate the man between feasts. **In these circumstances, it is an act of giving and sharing.** It can keep a relationship alive and can be enjoyable to both partners.

Sadly, in some situations sexual intercourse is not possible. Some men may develop severe prostatitis and ejaculation can be very painful. Similarly, some women can find the sex act too painful. In these situations, masturbation of the partner should be considered. Fortunately, these circumstances are uncommon. **Indeed, some patients find orgasm as the one activity that totally relieves their symptoms.** This is probably because of the release of adrenaline and endorphins, but unfortunately the effects are short-lived and much energy is consumed in the process. Yet, sex is important for all relationships and should have a high priority because of its great benefits.

SUMMARY

1. Patients need to develop a strategy for understanding energy. They should think of: energy as money; losing energy, gaining energy, and making energy last.

2. PVFS patients need to use only the energy (money) that they have.

3. The cause of tiredness is not unfitness, but that PVFS has resulted in the body not behaving in a normal manner. The patient is ill.

4. Different types of activity use more/less energy. Activities may result in symptoms days later.

5. Relationships are emotional and use up energy through mental activity. They also create much stress. The amount of stress and energy varies with the type of relationship.

6. Patients may need to lose all of their friends before they can get better.

7. Relatives can be supportive. Some older parents may

be unduly demanding on patients. Patients should not feel guilty about their parents.

8. The family unit can determine whether a patient recovers. The patient's role within the family will have to change and help will have to be accepted.

9. Partners have an almost impossible task. For relationships to survive, several characteristics are necessary with sexual activity being the most difficult. Couples need to rethink their attitudes and to experiment in their sexual activities.

CHAPTER EIGHT

FOURTH STEP: GAINING ENERGY: SLEEP AND UNWIND

It was the best restaurant in the country. The dining-room was small and intimate. The atmosphere was perfect: the tables were not too close together and the lighting allowed you to see the food. But even better, the food was good and the restaurant had consistently won all the top awards for the last 10 years. Inevitably, it was expensive. No, it was very, very expensive. Nevertheless, it seemed just the place to see Ann Woods, a businesswoman who had built up her company over 20 years so that it now employed 500 people.

The chauffeur had parked the Mercedes and Ann was sitting at the best table in the restaurant. She had just ordered the most expensive meal on the menu and each course was accompanied by the finest wines. Just then, a friend who was leaving saw Ann and was obviously surprised at seeing her alone.

"It's my 25th wedding anniversary" replied Ann.

Her friend was in a hurry and did not want to pursue matters, but added:

"How are you?"

"I am fine" replied Ann "But business is bad. I am nearly bankrupt".

Her friend was a bit taken aback and said:

"Oh come on Ann! It can't be all bad. You are in the best restaurant in the country. You have just ordered the most expensive meal with the finest wines. On top of it all, your marriage has lasted 25 years despite all the difficulties of your running your own business. Most women would be content with what you have got."

Ann shook her head and ruefully replied:

"Yes, but last year I could afford to bring my husband."

Sleep and the ability to unwind are a bit like a loyal husband – easily forgotten during the celebration, and conveniently left at home. Sadly, the most important part of an individual can be taken for granted. Yet, to sleep and unwind are two essential skills for living in the modern world. Both can be elusive. The western world is full of people who cannot sleep; and our emphasis on physical activities can mean that many are unable to unwind. This is so sad. How can two natural body functions become unattainable goals?

The answer is simple: **we take sleep and the ability to unwind for granted.** Many have not been taught the ability to sleep and unwind. Both are necessary skills which take time to acquire, and much practice is required for one to become proficient. In schools of the future, they will be as important as learning how to cook. **PVFS patients need to know that sleep and the ability to unwind gain energy** (Figure 19). The more energy that is gained in this way, the more energy is available for physical and mental activities.

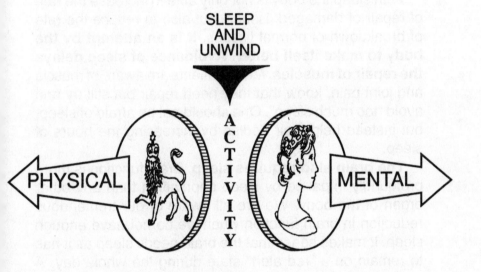

SLEEP AND UNWIND

ACTIVITY

PHYSICAL

MENTAL

Figure 19   The ten-pence coin
Sleep and the ability to unwind earn money. The two sides of the ten-pence coin show how money (energy) is spent. The lion represents physical activity, and equally the head represents mental activity.

113

SLEEP

Sleep has been described as the great restorer of the body. During the day, the body breaks down tissues faster than they can be renewed; whereas at night, the process of renewal is greater. **There is not only physical repair of muscles, but the brain also requires time for renewal and reorganisation of information acquired during the day.**

With sleep the body is not only able to increase the rate of repair of damaged tissues, but also to reduce the rate of breakdown of normal tissues. **It is an attempt by the body to make itself better. Avoidance of sleep delays the repair of muscles.** Many patients are aware of muscle and joint pain, know that they need repair but still try and avoid "too much sleep". One should not be afraid of sleep, but instead help their bodies by increasing the hours of sleep.

The brain also requires sleep. Brain function is more profoundly impaired by sleep deprivation than any other organ of the body. We are all aware of our tremendous reduction in brain function when we do not have enough sleep. It makes sense that the brain needs sleep as it has to remain on a "red alert" state during the whole day. A period of repair of the brain circuits and reassessment of the day's events is essential preparation for the new day. **Therefore, sleep can be curative.** It may be helpful to remember Shakespeare's words of Macbeth:

"Sleep that knits up the ravell'd sleave of care,
The death of each day's life, sore labour's bath,
Balm of hurt minds, great nature's second course,
Chief nourisher in life's feast."

SLEEP MYTHS

The public perceives good sleep to be: instant sleep as the head touches the pillow; total unconsciousness for eight hours; no vivid dreams; and awakening totally refreshed. **This perception of sleep is too simple and is inaccurate in many ways.** For PVFS patients, they need to learn the truth about sleep and get rid of many of their false perceptions. As sleep is so important, some popular myths must be carefully considered:

Awakening during the night
It is considered to be very poor sleep if one wakes often during the night. It is not recognised that this concept of sleep has been learnt: babies do not sleep through the night, and in terms of survival it makes more sense to wake frequently. Sleeping throughout the night is learned behaviour designed for modern living; and with illness, there is often reversion to a more natural sleeping pattern with frequent awakening.

Length of sleep
Most people have 7-8 hours sleep per night, with some needing 6 hours and others 9 hours. However, there are also tremendous differences with age: a baby of two months sleeps 18 hours, a three-year old for 13 hours, a twenty-five year old for 8 hours and a seventy-five year old for 5 hours. In addition, **centuries ago, people were able to vary their sleeping hours with the seasons of the year.** Thus in winter, they would sleep 14-16 hours and thus have less need for food, warmth or light. Whilst in the summer, they would sleep 4-6 hours and make use of the daylight. Today, how many people would be able to

115

do this? Indeed, many patients believe more or less than 8 hours sleep per night is "abnormal"!

A constant complaint of patients is the increased amount of sleep that they require. For some, double the sleeping time still does not seem to be enough. Others try to stop themselves sleeping as they fear "sleeping their lives away". It is important to realise that there is a reason for sleep: their bodies are trying to repair damage. **Sleep, unlike fat, is not stored in the body.** The analogy with fat is instructive. Many patients only experience of being responsible for their own health is in the control of their weight. To remove fat one stops eating. Thus, it seems logical if one sleeps too much, to stop sleeping. **But, one sleeps to recover from the past and not to prepare for the future.**

Restrictions on sleep make matters worse. **A catastrophic double mistake is if a patient decides to "snap" out of his condition by excessive exercise and reduced sleep.** This is like getting a £10,000 loan to repay a debt, burning the money and wondering why there is no improvement in the financial position. **During sleep, there is healing of damaged body tissues.**

Vivid dreams
Everyone dreams every night. Many people do not realise that they need to dream every night. If this is prevented by awakening individuals as they start to dream, these individuals develop severe psychological symptoms. In some societies, talking and remembering dreams are an important part of the day. However, in the West, we have been taught to forget our dreams. When faced with a child having had a vivid dream, parents often say, "Never mind, go to sleep and forget the dream."

116

Similarly, "It was only a dream, think of something else". The teaching to the child is that dreams are not important and should be forgotten. In PVFS, vivid dreams are common and are normal and should not be a source of worry.

Terrible sleep

If patients do not understand sleep cycles, they frequently complain of terrible sleep. There are natural cycles at 20-30 minutes and at 90 minutes. If patients awake at these times, they feel refreshed. However, if patients awake at 60 minutes, they may be in the deepest stage of sleep. This is when a sleeper is "dead to the world" and ignores outside stimulation such as a telephone ringing. If patients awake at this stage, **they feel terrible and not refreshed so many become convinced that sleep makes them worse.**

Night into day

Very many patients get into the habit of getting up late, watching too much television and going to bed late. They end up sleeping during the day and staying up all night. **This is a similar position to individuals who have jet-lag or are working a night shift.** It is perhaps complicated by the natural biological clock which works a 25-hour day, so there is a natural inclination to turn night into day. This inclination has to be corrected by frequent adjustments to our 24-hour day such as work, radio, television, etc.

Re-adjusting the body clock back to normal is not easy. **The answer is that patients have to go to bed 3 hours later each "night" and get up 3 hours later each "morning".** After a few days, patients can go to bed and get up at a chosen time. They must now stick to this new schedule. Any late nights and they will have to repeat the treatment all over again.

NAPS

There is a range of opinion on naps or short sleeps. Many feel that only the lazy members of society need to take naps, and the strong do not need such time-outs. There is also the image of the overweight Pickwickian character who eats and sleeps all of the time. Another strong image is of elderly people who are always falling asleep in front of the television or when there are visitors. There is no doubt **in Britain that naps are assigned to the lazy, overweight or elderly.**

In southern Europe, the position is quite different. **The siesta is part of the life-style and culture.** These naps after lunch reflect the sleepiness after eating and the hot midday temperatures. However, a great advantage is that it allows individuals to stay up longer at night. Many feel that the body's natural internal sleep-wake clock is designed for two sleeps a day (a short one in the afternoon and a long one at night).

Many patients who are unaccustomed to naps can find them daunting. A feeling of being a zombie after a nap is usually due to the individual getting up in the wrong part of the sleep cycle. In addition, **it takes time to learn to nap** and patients often do not feel real benefit until 2-3 months later. Like all great skills, much effort is required for one to become proficient.

Another common argument against naps is that if there is a sleep during the day, the person would not be able to sleep at night. Again there is some truth in this, but there is also some benefit. In PVFS patients, the total sleep for a 24-hour period has to be increased, so if one slept during the day, there is a smaller requirement in the night sleep. However, it also **takes time to adjust to two sleeps per day.**

Very many great world leaders have been addicted to naps. Winston Churchill and Margaret Thatcher are two excellent examples. The message is clear: **when you have very little time for sleep, naps are a great bonus.** It is a valuable lesson to PVFS patients. Naps gain time and energy.

INSOMNIA

Many patients have difficulty sleeping because of several common problems:

1. Symptoms. A host of symptoms can easily interfere with a good night's sleep. Hotness or coldness, twitching muscles, muscle cramps, muscle and joint pains, itching and numbness of arms or legs are the most common complaints. With all of these symptoms, it **is important not to become annoyed or angry with being woken up.** It is best to adopt an attitude of being woken up by a mischievous child or pet, and try to get back to sleep. Leg muscle cramps are worrying, but pulling the toes towards the shin is usually effective. It is worth doing this several times before you go to sleep as it may prevent cramps developing.

2. Active mind. An active mind which is unable to switch off and go to sleep is commonly found. Many patients complain that they feel physically exhausted but cannot stop their mind thinking and worrying. **It is critical that patients develop the ability to blank their mind out.** It is best to do an "unwind exercise". This is considered in more detail in the "Unwind" section of this chapter.

3. Early awakening. Another common complaint is to wake after a few hours sleep and not be able to go back to sleep.

A quick return to sleep depends on an adoption of an unwind exercise and not doing more thinking. The most common mistake is to start thinking and become worried, anxious and wide awake. When this happens, it can help to get out of bed, have a drink of water and then return to bed and go through an unwind exercise.

A few patients have early morning awakening. This is often when patients are agitated or anxious. It might be accompanied by depression. The best remedy is to deal with the anxiety or depression, and then sleep will return to normal.

AIDS TO SLEEP

Boredom, warmth and satisfaction of bodily needs are the best combination for good sleep. Other aids are:

1. Regular sleeping times. Going to bed and awakening at the same time each day is very helpful for good sleep.

2. No external stimuli. Noises, television and radio do not help going to sleep. Draughts, wind, rattling radiators can all interfere with sleep.

3. Bed-time snacks. It is not a good idea to eat or drink too much before bed. Malted, milky drinks (such as Horlicks or Ovaltine) help sleep; whereas tea and coffee are stimulants and interfere with sleep. Excessive alcohol is also not a good idea.

UNWIND

In the modern world, people have to be "keyed up" and "ready to go". It is therefore not surprising that many people are "wound up" at the end of the day. These people need to "unwind" as a full life involves movement between these two states: **a person needs to be wound up at certain times and unwound** at others. Sadly, whilst most people are able to wind themselves up, only a minority are able to unwind. **Many PVFS patients need to learn to unwind.** Why have I chosen to use the word **"unwind"** instead of **"relaxation"**? Both of these words have similar meanings, however, there are important differences. Firstly, relaxation is usually more associated with muscles, for example "make less rigid", whereas I am more concerned with the relaxation of the mind. Secondly, relaxation is often associated with "recreation". Although the concept of re-creating (or "making again") is consistent with my views, other interpretations of recreation (such as "interval of free time") are not the objectives that I have. Lastly, "unwind" epitomises my approach of "undoing", "unravelling" or "disentangling" life's problems.

Relaxation is often used to mean "not being active", "sitting in front of the television", "resting", or "recreation". Many patients think that this can do them good. Indeed they quickly remind others how this compared with what they did previously. Unfortunately, **sitting in front of a television rarely does anyone a lot of good.** PVFS patients have to learn to unwind. **To unwind is an active process which creates energy and allows patients to recharge their batteries.**

A special unwind technique, **EMBME**, has been developed for PVFS patients. This technique is described in detail ("Unwind! Understand and control life, be better!!" by Dr Darrel Ho-Yen, Dodona Books, 1991 ISBN 0-9511090-0-2-2). This book shows how the skill of unwinding can deal with the stress in modern life.

The unwind technique has five stages:

i)   **Entrance** requires that enough time should be set aside, there should be mental commitment, a quiet comfortable place and enough concentration.

ii)   **Muscles:** With the patient lying down or sitting in a comfortable chair, there is gradual contraction and relaxation of the muscles in the legs, abdomen, arms, shoulders and face.

iii)   **Breathing:** Breathe in fully and breathe out fully. Repeat this three times and then breathe naturally. Count up to fifty and then proceed to the next stage.

iv)   **Mind control:** This stage unwinds the mind by concentrating on a peaceful scene (such as a tree, beach, lake or mountain) in your imagination with your eyes closed. Remove any unwanted thoughts. Repetition of the word EBMBE again and again can help.

v) **Exit.** Open your eyes slowly, appreciate your surroundings and yawn. Stretch arms and legs. Slowly get up. Shout "EMBME!"

Best results from unwinding are obtained when an individual has two half hour sessions each day. At times of stress, there should be four sessions per day (morning and evenings). **Remember that it takes time to learn to unwind.** Most people take several months before there is great benefit, but some can get an immediate boost to their energy levels.

DAILY DIARY

Sleep and unwind sessions are two very important parts of the daily diary. Patients should **record the total number of hours in a 24-hour day that they are lying down in bed with their eyes closed and with no noise in the room.** I do not mind if patients are not asleep. However, it is critical that there is no noise in the room. It is also important that patients try and not think or worry. If sleep is in several periods during the day, record only the total amount for the day.

The diary of patients who are still at work frequently show a pattern of 6-7 hours sleep from Monday to Friday, and 11-12 hours sleep on Saturday/Sunday. Obviously **the patient was suffering from sleep deficit during the week and making up for this at weekends.** The way forward is to agree that the minimum sleep each night from Monday to Friday is 7 hours, and the minimum for Saturday/Sunday is 12 hours. **This simple change can produce dramatic changes in scores.**

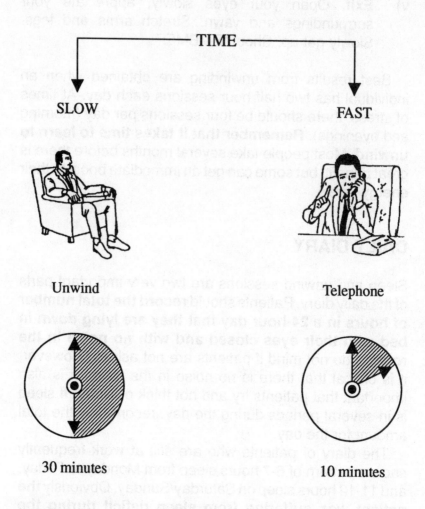

Figure 20 Time

When patients are performing unwind, time goes slowly and 30 minutes may appear to be 1 hour. However, when they are on the telephone, time goes fast and 1 hour appears to be 10 minutes. Patients should spend no more than 10 minutes on one telephone call.

124

Unwind sessions are very important and each session should be recorded, eg unwind x 2. Ideally, **a patient should have at least two sessions per day.** As this is a means of gaining extra energy, it is particularly useful before periods of increased demands, for example on the day before a night out. It is better before the event than after.

Time goes slowly when patients are having an unwind session (Figure 20). This is because many are bored. However, when on the telephone, patients are stimulated and time goes fast. Patients prefer to be on the telephone but an unwind session is more beneficial.

SUMMARY

1. PVFS patients need to learn to sleep and unwind to gain energy.

2. Sleep is necessary for muscle and brain renewal, and proper functioning. Sleep is curative.

3. There are many sleep myths such as awakening during night, length of sleep, vivid dreams, terrible sleep and turning night into day.

4. Naps allow people to be refreshed during the day and reduce the overall requirement for sleep.

5. Insomnia is caused by many factors (especially patients' symptoms, an active mind and early awakening). Patients should take appropriate action.

6. There are many aids to sleep, especially regular sleeping times, no external stimuli and bed-time snacks.

7. The ability to unwind must be learnt. The technique

EMBME is a major skill which aids recovery.

8. The daily diary must include total hours a patient is in bed with their eyes closed with no noise in the room. Unwind sessions should be twice daily and the number recorded.

CHAPTER NINE

FIFTH STEP:
MAKING ENERGY LAST

Dan was a studious young man who approached life in a methodical manner. He always had a plan. After College, he had a flying start with a stock-broking firm dealing with volatile shares. Dan's charm and selling ability did him proud. Soon, he had an expensive flat and car. Then, the market collapsed and Dan was made redundant. Bad luck was replaced by more bad luck. Months went by but his optimism remained.

One day he met an old man in the park and they got talking. Dan explained:

"I've asked for money, begged for money and even cried for money".

The old man was not impressed and asked:

"Have you tried working for it?"

"Good heavens! No!" Dan replied "I'm in a bad position, but I'm still sticking to my game plan. I have a while to go before I consider work."

The old man could not believe his ears:

"You cannot be serious! Work is the only way!"

"Maybe", replied Dan "But my plan is to go through the alphabet, and it will take some time before I get to "w".

Very many PVFS patients are like Dan and do not want to work at making energy last. To many onlookers, it seems an easy solution to their problem. However, for patients, it will take some time before they consider the great benefits of making energy last. **Instead, they are happier to ask, beg and cry for good health.** If patients would like to **work** at making energy last, there are simple rules: go slow; never do two things at once; have boredom periods; save little bits; choose type of activity; and enjoy good scores. Although these rules are simple, **for PVFS patients they are extremely difficult as this involves facing the truth of their situation and taking appropriate action.** Like much of life, it can be easier to be dishonest with oneself than face the truth.

Two good examples from life may also help. When people lose their job, it can be a long time before they adjust to their reduced circumstances. Instead, they continue to spend as before, hoping to be employed soon. **The position is similar to PVFS patients, and as with unemployment, those individuals who adjust best, do so early.** Patients need to live within their budget (energy and money) now.

Another example emphasises the need to develop skills. If one gave a group of people £10 each to spend on food for a week, there would be a variety of responses. Some would not be able to feed themselves for one day; others would be able to eat for two weeks. Similarly, PVFS patients have to learn the skill of making money (energy) last.

GO SLOW

I once had a teacher who went through life in three speeds:

slow, dead slow and stop. Everyone ridiculed him. Yet, he was one of the most well-adjusted individuals that I have known. He recognised that rushing around is a great waste of energy. I am always saddened when I walk down a corridor with a patient and the patient is walking faster than I. It is as though he/she has something to prove. Patients are ill so why do they want to walk faster? Some hospitals insist that patients should be in wheelchairs. It is sensible. So **why do some patients abhor the suggestion that they should use a wheelchair?**

To me, it seems sensible that if you do not have a lot of energy, you do not spend what you have in walking. Worse, to try and walk faster than normal people seems to be particularly daft. Also, **how can people believe that you are ill if you behave as an Olympian?** Again and again, PVFS patients must recognise that they will be treated by the general public as they behave. **It is not unfair to be judged by your actions.**

NEVER DO TWO THINGS AT ONCE

An American President was once described as someone who could not chew gum and walk at the same time. It was a tremendous joke and produced much hilarity. No one bothered to consider how someone who was an American President could achieve so much whilst being so incapable. For PVFS patients, **it makes great sense never to do two things at once.** Working people have breakfast, read the papers and listen to the radio or television at the same time, all in 30 minutes. **This uses up a lot of energy as it requires a lot of concentration. For PVFS patients, these should be separate activities.**

Thus, patients should have breakfast (30 minutes), make coffee and drink it slowly (30 minutes), read the papers (30 minutes) and then listen to the radio or television (30 minutes). **What previously took 30 minutes should now take 2 hours; it uses less energy and makes available resources last.** In addition, one and a half more hours have been used up.

BOREDOM PERIODS

"To bore" means "To tire by being dull, repetitious or uninteresting". It is what most PVFS patients detest – the last thing that they would want to do. Over the last years, the **greatest change in my management technique is to recommend boredom periods.** Why? Because if one is bored, then one is using less energy. When we are stimulated and excited, adrenaline flows and we use maximum energy. Is it not better to be bored and wanting to go to sleep?

Most patients answer this question by saying that if they were bored all day, they would become depressed ... and that would be even worse! I agree. So the answer is to have **both boredom and excitement, and also lose less energy.** How can this be achieved?

It can be achieved by breaking the day up into half hour periods (Figure 21). For example, if you would like to watch television, precede this period with a boredom period and after the half-hour of television have another boredom period. **Whilst you are being bored, try and look forward to your indulgence – a period of television.** In this way, you will probably find that you will enjoy the television even more than normal. The end result is you

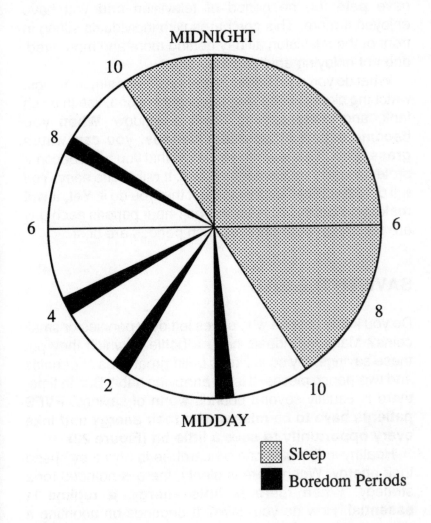

MIDNIGHT

10

8

6

6

8

4

2

10

MIDDAY

- Sleep
- Boredom Periods

Figure 21 Ideal day
The ideal day is broken up into many half-hour slots, with lots of boredom periods.

have **paid** for the period of television **and** you have enjoyed it more. This compares with individuals sitting in front of the television all day getting more and more tired, and not enjoying anything they see.

What do you do in boredom periods? I like simple things: watching clouds in the sky, trees in the wood, fish in a fish tank, and water running down a window. **When you become expert at boredom periods, you can watch grass grow.** This is when you know that you have become professional at making energy last. It will not be easy. You will detest yourself every moment that you do it. **Yet, it will make you better!** At least two half-hour periods each day are recommended, but four such periods are best.

SAVE LITTLE BITS

Do you know anyone who saves left over pennies or small coins? Many individuals have a bottle in which they put these savings. My sons like to build great piles of pennies and two-pence pieces. It is an annoying habit. But, in time, there is usually several pounds worth of savings. **PVFS patients have to be misers with their energy and take every opportunity to save a little bit (Figure 22).**

Healthy individuals can be carefree in how they spend their energy. When there is plenty, there is no need for a strategy. **When there is little energy, a regime is essential.** How do you save? It depends on adopting a different mental attitude. Instead of trying to finish the gardening, you stop early when the job is half done. You plan to stay two hours at the party, but leave 10 minutes early. You say someone can visit for an hour and insist that they leave after an hour and five minutes, instead

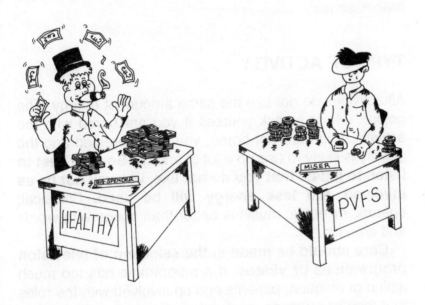

Figure 22 Big spender and miser
Healthy individuals are big spenders and can throw away pound notes.
Whereas PVFS patients must be misers with their money (energy),
and count every coin.

allowing them to stay for 2 hours. You plan to go shopping for one hour, but come home after 50 minutes.

Every little bit of energy that is saved is there for tomorrow. More importantly, it means that you do not have to borrow energy today. If you do not have to go into your reserves, it means that your body has more energy to heal itself now. **If the body can start to heal itself now, it is obvious that you will get better faster.** It simply makes sense.

TYPE OF ACTIVITY

All activities do not use the same amount of energy. The golden rule is to ask yourself if you are bored with the activity. If you are not bored, you are interested and the activity is likely to use up a lot of energy. **So, it is best to listen to music that you do not like, you will not be as involved and less energy will be used.** Classical, operatic or ethnic music is better than songs with words and emotion.

Care should be made in the selection of television programmes or videos. If a programme has too much action or emotion, patients end up involved with the roles that they see with as much adrenaline being released as the actors. Love stories and drama are particularly good at using up energy. Nature, travel or cooking programmes are good at using up very little energy. Indeed, two hours of a cooking programme uses as much energy as half an hour of an emotional, daily soap programme. **A good idea is to decide on the type of programme based on your scores.**

Activities such as watching fish in a fish tank or a pet

playing with itself are good at making energy last. Although pets can be a great help to recovery, large dogs that need daily exercise are not. **The cat which looks after itself is a much better role model for a patient.** Indeed, if patients can adopt the single-mindedness of a cat, recovery is assured.

ENJOY GOOD SCORES

When you get a good score in your diary, it should be enjoyed. Like receiving a certificate, **one should take some time and just look at the accomplishment.** The diary is designed for the scores to have a separate page so that progress can be visually appreciated.

Patients should also enjoy the feel of the score. Scores are not what you can do, **but what you feel that you can do.** Sadly, some patients have a negative response to a good score. There is disbelief followed by the thought that the score is only true if the individual could do more. They then try to do activities representing the score. When there is the predictable relapse, the patient's retort is that it shows that the score was not real. It is a powerful self-fulfilling prophecy.

The daily diary is not only a source of information but also encouragement. The low scores give warning that there is too much activity. **The high scores are an accolade of good practice.** As the high scores have been hard won, they should be treasured. Then, high scores can produce more high scores and success follows.

SUMMARY

1. Patients have to be prepared to work at making energy last. Much has to be learnt and put into practice.

2. Patients must slow their lives down. Their ability to do this will aid recovery but also make others recognise that they are ill.

3. Never do two things at once. It takes more energy and means there is more time in the day to fill.

4. There should be regular boredom periods every day. At least two half-hour periods are needed, but four such periods are best.

5. Patients have to be misers with their energy, and take every opportunity to save a little bit of energy.

6. Activities have to be carefully assessed as some use more energy than others. The activity chosen should depend on your score.

7. Good scores should be treasured and enjoyed. They represent an accolade of good practice.

CHAPTER TEN
FOOD AND DIETS

"Let food be your medicine and medicine your food".

This advice is attributed to Hippocrates, a Greek physician who practised medicine some 400 years before the birth of Christ. For his many writings and accurate observations, he has been called the "Father of Medicine". But perhaps the best indication of the high regard his fellow doctors had for him, was the adoption of his medical ethics in the "Hippocratic Oath" which is taken by every doctor on graduation.

The health properties of food have been recognised for thousands of years. The slaves who were assigned to building the giant pyramids were given daily doses of garlic to prevent illness. Subsequently, the Roman Empire is said to have survived without doctors with the help of the common cabbage. This lowly vegetable has great nutritional properties apart from being a useful wound dressing.

For PVFS patients, some understanding of food and diets is important but not essential. **Too many patients spend too much time worrying about food and diets.** For those with particularly worrying abdominal complaints, especially those who have been ill for many years, the section on diets may help.

FOOD

Health is made up of the triad of activity, food and sleep (Figure 23). **Matters are changed with illness when food is required for healing rather than activity.** It is important for all ill patients to have sufficient protein (meat, chicken, fish), carbohydrates (bread, rice), vitamins and minerals (vegetables and fruits). Fortunately, most patients living as part of a family are likely to eat well. **Small more frequent meals and eating the major meal in the middle of the day can also be particularly helpful.**

Patients who have been ill under one year should not worry about diets. This cannot be emphasised too much. Too many patients waste great amounts of energy and money on diets. It is as if they cannot get tablets to cure their disease so they become diet-fixated. Instead, they should simply attempt to eat normally. Problems are likely to occur when patients live alone because there is the temptation to miss meals. Patients often say that they are not hungry and have no energy to cook. After some weeks, the less you eat, the less you want to eat. **If a patient is not eating normally then major problems may arise, including anorexia nervosa.** Sadly, this is becoming more and more common among young women patients.

Vitamins are present in fresh fruit and vegetables. Vitamin tablets may be purchased and can be expensive. Patients often feel the need to take extra vitamins, not unlike buying a "tonic". **Most patients do not require**

HEALTH

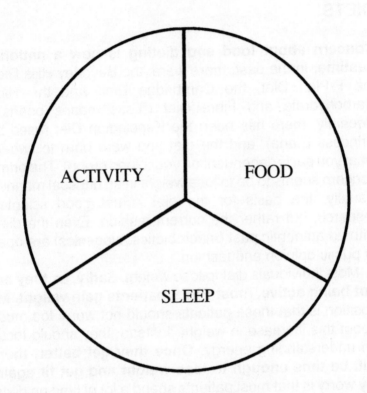

ACTIVITY

FOOD

SLEEP

Figure 23   Health
For a healthy life, there are three main requirements: activity to occupy
your time; food for your daily activities; and sufficient sleep for your
body. Many patients spend too much energy on food compared to
their activities and sleep.

extra vitamins and much money can be saved. Patients who are living alone and not eating normally may benefit from extra vitamins.

DIETS

Concern about food and dieting is now a national pastime. In the past, there were: the Beverley Hills Diet, the F-Plan Diet, the Cambridge Diet, and the High Carbohydrate and Fibre Diet ("Less means beans"). Recently, there has been the Kensington Diet (used by Princess Diana), and the diet you were born to (where what you eat is dependent on your blood group). The prime concern seems to be to lose weight in an unusual manner. Usually, the basis for the diet is not good scientific research, but rather the current fashion. Even the diets with an authentic past (macrobiotics, biogenics) are open to public opinion and fashion.

Most individuals diet to lose weight. **Sadly, as they are not being active, most PVFS patients gain weight.** My position is that these patients should not worry too much about this increase in weight. Instead, they should focus on understanding energy. **Once they get better, there will be time enough to lose weight and get fit again.** My worry is that most patients spend a lot of time on diets, and do not try to understand energy which is much harder to do. If patients are very worried about gaining weight, **the most effective solution is to eat less.** As they are not being as active, this is the best solution.

For patients with severe abdominal complaints or illness for many years, they diet to feel better. Sadly, there are many available diets, and some of these diets require large amounts of time (Figure 24). **If you cannot find the time and energy to eat normally, you do not have sufficient time or energy for a diet.** The **anticandida** diets have many advocates. They are very time-consuming and can be quite expensive. I do **not** feel that most patients benefit from this diet. **I would rather patients take the time and effort to understand energy.** In my experience, this understanding is far more likely to produce recovery.

The diet that I have found most helpful to patients is the **"Hay System"**. This is superbly explained in "Food Combining for Health" by Doris Grant and Jean Joice (1984, Thorsons). Recently there have been many other books which have been published which deal with food combining. However, the message is similar. There are five major rules:

a) starches and sugars should not be eaten with proteins and acid fruits at the same meal
b) vegetables, salads and fruits should form the major part of the diet
c) proteins, starches and fats should be eaten in small quantities
d) refined, processed foods should be avoided
e) an interval of 4-5 hours should elapse between meals of different character.

How does the Hay System work in PVFS patients? Complete answers are not available. However, in patients with severe abdominal complaints or long illness, it is likely that the gastrointestinal tract is affected with disease. **The Hay System reduces the workload for a patient with gastrointestinal dysfunction.** Whereas an unaffected

141

TIME FOR FOOD

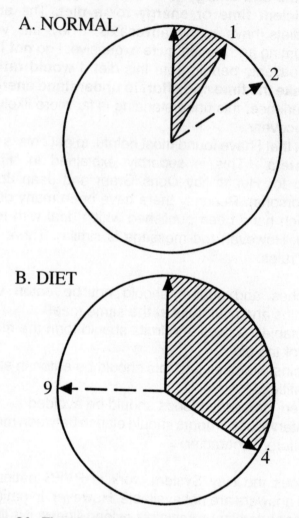

A. NORMAL

B. DIET

Figure 24   Time for food
The normal individual usually spends between 1-2 hours per day
preparing and consuming food. For those on diets, this time is greatly
increased to 4 hours and can be as much as 9 hours. Before starting
a diet, the time required should be carefully calculated.

gastrointestinal tract can easily cope with whatever is ingested, it makes sense to combine foods with similar digestive requirements when there is abnormal function of the gastrointestinal tract.

FOOD ALLERGIES

After a viral infection, patients may develop food allergies (British Medical Journal, 1981; 283: 1086) which can result in severe and worrying symptoms. The vast majority of PVFS patients do **not** have food allergies. **Food allergy is the immediate reaction to tiny amounts of a specific food.** It is often a life-long problem and total avoidance of the specific food is the main treatment.

Food allergies can produce similar complaints to those of PVFS. This is not surprising as both may be caused by abnormalities in the immune system. The situation is further complicated as PVFS patients can develop food allergies, and symptoms may be due to either. Fortunately, it is possible to separate the two conditions by testing for food allergies. **If symptoms are due to food allergies, they will go away when the causative food is avoided.** If symptoms are due to PVFS, they will not go away with a change of diet. Instead, only the slow recovery from the viral infection will see the disappearance of the complaints.

Tests
The simplest method of testing is the exclusion diet.
Over a period of weeks, various foods or groups of foods are introduced into the diet and their effects observed. If there is no adverse effect, the food is excluded as a

possible cause of the symptom. Ideally, the patient should start with a **5-day fast,** however, as this is very difficult for working people, it is more appropriate for those being tested in hospital. **An alternative start is to eat pork (or fish) for 3 meals a day for 5 days.** During this time no other food is eaten. As much spring water (bottled Malvern water) as desired can be drunk, but tap water is avoided (because of impurities, especially chlorine).

After the 5 days, a suspected food is eaten by itself instead of the evening meal (if a drink is to be tested, it is drunk after the usual meal of pork or fish). **If the food is causing an allergy, symptoms return within a few hours.** In this way, different foods and drink are slowly incriminated or excluded. Records must be detailed and all food taken every day must be recorded. If one particular food produces a severe reaction, the testing should not stop as that patient may be allergic to more than one food or group of foods.

Severe reactions may be stopped by drinking a tablespoon of sodium bicarbonate (bicarbonate of soda) in a half-pint of warm water. The sodium bicarbonate produces diarrhoea and so gets rid of the offending food. The theory behind starting with 5 days of meat (Cave Man diet) is that man has been eating meat for thousands of years and it is thus less likely to cause allergy. Whereas, only much later did man start to eat cereals and sugars and so these are more likely to cause allergy.

Hospital testing is more complete, but unfortunately there are few of these specialised units. Patients are starved for 5-days, but during this time they can drink as much spring water as they want. **If there is no improvement after the 5 days, the patient does not have a food allergy.** Improvement in symptoms suggest food allergy and the patient is then tested with one new food a day. Foods are sequentially tested, for example: sugars; cereals and grains (including wheat, rye, barley, oats, maize and rice); milk and milk products; eggs; chocolate and processed foods. Beverages (especially instant coffee, tea and chocolate) are then tested. Alcohol (except beer and whisky in grain-sensitive individuals) and tobacco are rare causes of allergy. In hospitals, other tests such as skin tests or testing of blood for particular IgE antibodies can also be performed.

The end result of testing is that patients should know they have a food allergy. **No improvement during the 5-day fast or the 5-day diet of pork implies that there is no food allergy.** If there is a food allergy, at the end of testing the patient should have a list of foods that produce symptoms. These foods can be confirmed as a cause of problems by **"challenging"**. This is the introduction of the food at a later date to see if symptoms are still produced. **Some patients find, after several months, that they are able to eat a particular food without side-effects when previously the same food produced symptoms.** Thus patients may need to rotate foods to adjust to symptoms developing or going away.

Pseudo-Food Allergy

This is when the patient has an underlying psychological problem rather than a food allergy (British Medical Journal, 1986; 292: 221-2). **The patient focuses on food allergy as the solution to his problems. There is an immediate placebo benefit from the exclusion of a particular food. However, it does not last.** To maintain improvement, there has to be continual placebo benefits from continual exclusion of foods. As this continues, there can be a serious risk of malnutrition and severe anorexia. This is another reason why patients should not undertake food allergy testing without first consulting their doctor. Early morning awakening, frequent changes in mood and disturbances in appetite and energy suggest an underlying psychological problem.

Commercial Allergy Testing

Facilities for testing for allergies in the National Health Service are limited. This has resulted in an increase in commercial allergy testing. A Consumer's Association "Which?" magazine survey, with the help of two London Hospitals (Lancet, 1987; i: 92-4), has **revealed many inadequacies in commercial tests.** They found that commercial tests on hair and blood were unable to detect some allergies; and, that there was poor reproducibility, i.e. when duplicate tests were sent there were different results. A worrying finding was that commercial tests reported many non-existent allergies. The tests are expensive and a decade later are still unreliable.

IgE antibodies (RAST) tests are available in most hospitals. There is national, external quality assessment of these tests; and, if local hospitals cannot do the tests, there should be no difficulty in arranging for another hospital to test the blood. The great advantage of these tests is that the results are reproducible in hospital laboratories throughout Britain.

FOOD INTOLERANCE

Food intolerance differs from food allergy in that with **food intolerance large quantities of the food are required**

146

and reactions are not immediate, occurring many hours later. The usual skin tests and laboratory tests which are used to diagnose food allergy are negative with food intolerance.

Diagnosis of food intolerance depends on demonstrating symptoms with exposure to the offending food. Patients should start with an exclusion diet as in excluding food allergy. Unlike food allergy, the reaction in food intolerance can be delayed and occur the next day. However, similar to food allergy, if symptoms do not improve on a 5 day diet of pork or fish, food intolerance is unlikely. **Food intolerance in PVFS patients is likely to be more common than food allergy.** Patients who are recently ill without abdominal complaints are unlikely to have food allergy or intolerance.

ALCOHOL

Alcohol intolerance is common in PVFS patients and may affect up to 30% of these patients. Alcohol can adversely affect PVFS patients in at least two ways. It may be part of a food allergy, alternatively it may be the direct action of alcohol. Surprisingly, it is not excessive alcohol intake (PVFS patients are rarely alcoholic), but moderate amounts that can have profound effects. Alcohol is a drug with a large number of actions on various tissues and organs in the body. For healthy people, the most noticeable action is on the brain. Inhibitions are removed and can result in hyperactivity. Another effect of alcohol is the dilatation of blood vessels which result in the feeling of warmth. **For many PVFS patients, there is usually profound tiredness and exhaustion after alcohol.**

SUMMARY

1. PVFS patients require a healthy diet as food is required for healing the body.

2. An understanding of food and diets is not necessary for all patients, but only those with severe abdominal complaints or illness for many years.

3. The diet that is the most useful is the Hay System and this can be adopted before food testing. This diet reduces the workload of the gastrointestinal tract.

4. Testing for food allergies or intolerance can be done in hospital or at home. Before starting such tests, patients should see their doctor, and carefully consider if they have the time and energy to test for allergies.

5. Patients do not have a food allergy or intolerance if they are not better after 5 days of fasting or 5 days of a pork (or fish) diet.

6. Many patients suffer adverse effects from small amounts of alcohol.

CHAPTER ELEVEN

EMPLOYMENT

Society puts pressure on its members to work, to be employed. Only through work by the majority can the society survive. There is an even greater pressure on individuals that through work can you only be happy. Samuel Johnson states the case: "Labour, if it were not necessary for the existence, would be dispensable for the happiness of man."

Few people realise that it is a game. There was the self-employed shop owner who was called up for jury service. When his name was called, he appeared before the judge and asked to be excused.

"I am very busy in this period before Christmas. Now, we make the profits for the whole year. Also I only employ one person, apart from my wife, to help."

"I see", remarked the judge "You are one of those people who feel that they are indispensable."

"No, your honour", replied the shop owner "I know that my wife and shop assistant can get along without me, but I don't want them to find out."

"Excused." said the judge.

Apart from its social status, employment has great emotional effects. With work, individuals feel that they are contributing to the community. They feel useful. They are playing their part. There is a sense of belonging, income, social contacts and purpose. It is a team game and these people are good to have on your team.

Suddenly, with PVFS, their role has been changed. Instead of a valuable member of the team, there is a handicapped one. Others have to do more work. The patient feels guilty. Not only is self-esteem lost, but also there is the realisation that they are helped, tolerated, even patronised. Illness is compounded by guilt and self-criticism. **Many feel that they are given a gun, and asked to do the honourable thing – shoot themselves.**

There is an excellent editorial in the British Medical Journal (1992; 305: 972) entitled **"Without work all life goes rotten."** Its message is clear: unemployment kills, ruins health and destroys families. It is not certain how unemployment kills, but it is probably a combination of the adoption of unhealthy behaviour, poverty, stress and a poor mental attitude to life. Walter Greenwood's "Love on the dole" (Penguin, 1969) has a superb quotation:

"Nothing to do with time; nothing to spend; nothing to do tomorrow nor the day after; nothing to wear; can't get married."

It all seems hopeless. **Yet, patients should remember that it is only a game.** Life has good bits and bad bits. Illness is a bad bit. If you cannot cope with the bad bits of life, you have not learnt to play the game of life. With illness, you have to concentrate on the major game of life which is not work, but survival. **Patients must remember that to survive and get better is the ultimate test.**

Ideally, individuals should enjoy their work and their

work should influence their health (Figure 25). **As this figure shows, many PVFS patients find themselves in the position where work results in a worsening of their health.** This is often because they are working inefficiently, and using a large amount of energy to achieve a mediocre result. Before they became unwell, they were able to do a job in 1 hour; with illness the same job may take 4 hours and have mistakes. **Less work (fewer hours) often results in the patient's health being improved.** The hours of work may also be more efficient and productive.

KEEPING A JOB

Most PVFS patients would have taken only a few days off work with their initial illness. Some would have taken no time off work. Going back to work is a test of "moral fibre"; those with low moral fibre have to have sick leave. Not only should there be an early return to work, "high achievers" make up for the time off when they return. In this way, **the patient is quickly exhausted and then the real problems begin.** The diagnosis of PVFS should not be made until the patient has been ill for 3 months. Fatigue for 2-3 months may rarely complicate many viral illnesses. Using a 3-month cut-off point is arbitrary, but it can be useful in separating those individuals who may take longer to recover.

After 3 months of being back at work, there is a predictable scenario. The patient is falling behind at work and sleeping a lot at home. **He is feeling unwell almost all of the time. There is difficulty concentrating. Bad decisions are being made.** He is a topic of conversation. The patient has a few days off, and then a few more. There

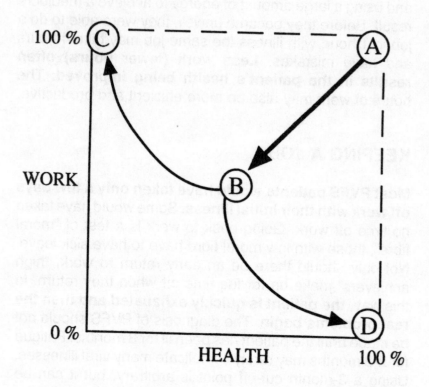

Figure 25 Work and health

At position A, full-time work has benefits on health. As work or health declines, the other is also reduced (B). From this position, some patients find that increasing work further reduces their health (C). Others may find that part-time work or unemployment allows their health to recover (D).

152

may be diarrhoea, blamed on the "take-away", and some more days are taken off work. He has become a regular visitor to his doctor. There are arguments with family and friends. What can be done?

At this stage, a patient has to answer a number of crucial questions. **How important is work to me? What would I do if I became unemployed? How would I feel?** This is a time for deciding on priorities. The most common mistake is for the patient to try and do everything. It cannot be done. Accustomed to having £10.00 to spend on sweets per day, there is now 10 pence and it has to last the whole week. **Patients cannot believe that life could have deteriorated so quickly.** There is a reluctance or an inability to see the situation objectively.

If patients want to remain employed, they have to be a miser with their energy. They have to:

a)   stop unnecessary exertion; if the job is physical, change the job.
b)   minimise all walking. **Walk slowly always.**
c)   think before any physical activity. Use the telephone.
d)   have a relaxation session or sleep at lunchtime.
e)   have a relaxation session or sleep as soon as work is finished.
f)   stop all social engagements.

All of the above seem excessive. It is. It has to be. PVFS patients who want to keep their job are asking a lot – there is nothing left over for anything else. If they want to do something else, they should give up the job. If all of the above are done, then there is a 95% chance of keeping the job. Most do not do all of the above. Most get away without losing their jobs. Most do not realise that all that they are doing is reducing their 95% chance to 70%, 50%, 30%, 10%....

Less time spent on social activities can also leave the brain free to concentrate on the job and home. Some have found that this honing down on the important things has produced more satisfaction at work and at home. At the start of the illness, both the brain and the muscles are easily exhausted. Brain function returns first and so it is possible to think normally after 2-3 months, provided that the patient is not too tired. **Indeed, a state where thinking compensates for activity, can produce better results.** Some have found promotion at work, purely because they use their time and energy more efficiently.

SICK LEAVE

As many patients can have a great benefit from the weekend or annual leave, **there is great optimism that a few weeks sick leave would allow them to recover.** Indeed, some patients would be willing to make a large bet that 6 weeks of rest would be accompanied by full recovery. **It does not happen.** The more usual pattern is that there is some benefit for the first two weeks, less benefit in the second two weeks and then anxiety and concern because of the lack of recovery in the last two weeks.

When a patient has a score of 4 or 5 out of 10 it is easier for a patient to stay at work than to benefit from sick leave. I believe that this is because PVFS patients are usually individuals who derive great satisfaction from work. Work is also normal and what they are accustomed to, whereas it takes some time to adjust to sick leave. **If patients feel that they need to have sick leave, they should plan for at least three months. In many cases, it is 6-9 months.** This is because there is great adrenaline which keeps individuals at work. When this stops, it takes the first month to adjust. There is benefit in the second month which can be consolidated in the last month. **A common trap is to substitute mental or social activities for work.** Patients who are not ready to return to work after six months have a major problem. This problem is usually that they have been unable to change their lifestyle. **They are unable to say "No!" to their friends and relatives, and are not in control of their lives.** They do not have an understanding of energy.

After the first six months of full pay, the next six months of half pay are a patient's last good chance of returning to work. **Matters are now desperate, but many patients fail to recognise their situation.** Somehow there appears to be great optimism, and the failures over the previous six months are not recognised. At this stage, it is possible for patients to return to work if they seriously adopt the five steps to recovery advocated in this book.

RETURN TO WORK

Patients should not try to return to work unless they score 8 out of 10 for a month. Occasionally, 7 out of 10 is acceptable. **Many patients are made worse by returning to work too early.** The job should not be too physical. Some patients are able to start with 2-3 half-days per week and build up. This is ideal, but a lot depends on the type of job and how the patient feels. Most patients are forced to return to half-time work. If a patient has scored 8 out of 10 for a month, this is very likely to be successful. **Patients need to think about returning to work for 1-2 months before they return.** Returning to work requires confidence. If a patient can think about the situations of work and how they may be coped with, confidence is built up. **It is not possible to suddenly decide on Friday night that you will start work on Monday morning.**

Many patients decide to return to part-time work by deciding on working two full days and one half-day, and resting four full days and one half-day. Although this seems acceptable, it is likely to fail. This is because in one full day it is possible to exhaust yourself so much that it takes one week to recover. As stated before, energy is obtained every day, so it is better to return to work as five half-days per week (Figure 26).

To increase your work from half-time to full-time also requires care. Usually, in the first two weeks, patients have difficulty in coping with the return to work. There is much need for relaxation and sleeping, with no social life. The diary may fall to 7, with an occasional 6 out of 10. After 2-3 weeks, the patient feels better and the diary scores return to 8 out of 10. **Before increasing work, scores should remain at 8 out of 10 for 1-2 weeks.**

Ideally, patients should increase working hours only every 6-8 weeks and providing that diary scores do not get worse. If scores fall to 5 out of 10, or less, hours should be reduced, as the patient is obviously not coping with work. For higher scores, work can be kept at the same hours. **Work should be increased every day by one hour.** Thus, patients should work their normal mornings, have their lunch break, and then work an additional hour every day. It is tempting to work a full five-

RETURN TO WORK

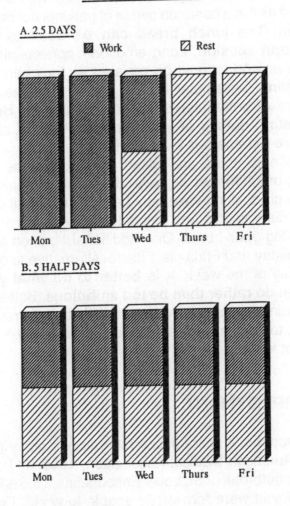

A. 2.5 DAYS

Work ▨   Rest ▨

Mon   Tues   Wed   Thurs   Fri

B. 5 HALF DAYS

Mon   Tues   Wed   Thurs   Fri

Figure 26 Return to work
It is tempting to return to part-time work by working 2.5 days, and resting the rest of the week (A). However, you may exhaust yourself in one full day so that you need a week to recover. It is better to work 5 half-days, either mornings or afternoons (B). This is less likely to totally exhaust you, and you are more likely to recover for the next day's work.

157

hour stretch each day and miss lunch. This should be resisted as it is a common cause of patients not being able to cope. **The lunch break can be used to have a relaxation session.** Long emotional conversations with people at work should be resisted as they can be very exhausting. Once patients have been ill for some months, they are of great interest to their colleagues. **However, recounting details of your illness or social chat can be more exhausting than working.**

Additional hours are added on in the same way as before, one hour per day over the week. In some cases, a more gradual increase may be indicated. It all depends on the diary scores and maintaining 7-8 out of 10 before increasing your hours. One additional hour on Monday, Wednesday and Friday is a useful alternative to one hour each day of the week. **It is better to do what you feel you can do rather than be too ambitious.** Better results are obtained more quickly if you make slow progress rather than do too much, have a relapse and have to reduce your hours of work.

UNEMPLOYMENT

This happens. It is not uncommon. In one study (Journal of the American Medical Association, 1938; 111: 15-17), after an outbreak of St. Louis Encephalitis, 16.5% of those unemployed were "physically unable to work". **For most patients, unemployment is not sudden, it is probably a product of several months of underperformance.** Many resign through pride, but a few are fired. Such an event, whether the patient jumped or was pushed, is a major life-event. Matters are made worse because PVFS patients were often good workers with an impressive work record. Comparable life-events can by themselves produce many of the symptoms of PVFS. The patient is on the ground and someone has put the boot in.

It is helpful to consider how this has happened. For many, it was because they tried to do too much. They were too ambitious. They exhausted themselves. Exhaustion is a powerful tool for disorientation. A person, disorientated and confused, can behave in an uncharacteristic way. They need time to recover, and to think. Unemployment becomes not so much a bad card in the game, but rather that the game has ended. For a few, it is just that their illness is so severe that it is incompatible with work. **For most, their own actions have produced an intolerable situation.**

Unemployment can be associated with excessive alcohol consumption, depression, suicide or attempted suicide (British Medical Journal, 1985; 291: 1563-6). Mortality is increased among the unemployed (British Medical Journal, 1987; 294: 86-90), but some of this may be due to greater cigarette consumption. **All of this ill-health adds to the problems associated with PVFS. It is a deep, deep pit.** There are two choices: either curl up in a corner, or try and claw a way out. The options are not easy.

But what a single, great opportunity!! There is time. Time to rest and recuperate. Time to think and plan. Not many people are given such an opportunity. Horace (65-8 BC) said: "Adversity has the effect of eliciting talents which in prosperous circumstances would have lain dormant." **The first great benefit, is that the patient rests.** Unfortunately, benefits may not result because a vast amount of energy can be lost on emotions. There is self-pity, often manifest by a withdrawing, a crying into the pillow, and a retreat into sleep. There is shock. Disbelief lasts weeks. In these weeks, there is greatly reduced activity. During this time the body tries to recover. Unfortunately, much energy is lost with mental activity. **Emotions are up and down; there is great mourning of the loss of a job.** These are common reactions for normal individuals, but everything is accentuated and made worse for PVFS patients.

Every patient needs to make the great decision to face life again. For some, this is impossible and they may not work again. For the brave, after 6-8 weeks, they attempt to find some answers. What has happened? Why did it happen? Why did I react like that? What do I want? What will make me happy? What can I get? The vast majority of the population do not have the time to consider such questions. Inscribed on the Temple of Apollo at Delphi, Greece, is a saying ascribed to the Seven Wise Men **"Know thyself"**. PVFS patients have this fantastic opportunity. Probably less than 5% of the population know themselves, and most who do not are dissatisfied with their job.

Loss of a job is like other great losses in life and is accompanied by a grieving process. **There are predictable stages and effects.** Yet, many feel that their experience is unique and others could not possibly understand their situation. Although this may be comforting for the patient, it is untrue. As I have had to deal with many patients with great losses (unemployment, end of relationships, failure at exams, financial ruin, betrayal etc) I wrote the book **"Climbing Out of the Pit of Life"**, Dodona Books, 1995 (ISBN 0-9511090-49). In this book, the ladder (**l**ifeless, **a**nger, **d**enial, **d**isgrace,

endeavour, renewal) **describes the stages of deep loss
and how to progress from each stage to the next.** It is
possible to climb out of the pit, and use the opportunity to
gain strength and happiness.

PVFS patients should be **honest** about their situation.
**They should decide how they want to live, and if they
are prepared to climb the difficult road to recovery.**
The plan advocated in this book is not easy. Many are
unable to change their lifestyle. Yet, I am always amazed
at how much can be achieved by a willingness to learn,
especially from past mistakes.

PART-TIME WORK

One feature of modern society is the greater opportunity
for part-time work. **For patients happy in their job, part-
time work can be an excellent solution.** It allows them
more time to rest. It is positive, as the decision is made in
the expectation that health will improve, and that a return
to full-time work will be possible. Fortunately, patients with
PVFS are often good employees, and employers are
usually sympathetic to such a temporary change.

**Like many other decisions for PVFS patients, it is
best if patients make the decision to do part-time work
before they are forced to by the illness.** Sadly, many
patients have financial demands which may preclude part-
time work. It is often only a reasonable alternative in those
families where both partners are at work. As with a return
to work, part-time work before full-time employment is
recommended. It allows time for the individual to adjust to
the demands of work.

For patients who have been unemployed, a new

part-time job is a possibility. However, part-time jobs are very dependant on the economic circumstances in the country. They may also be very physically demanding or very stressful; such jobs must be avoided. Taking **any** job is always a weak position from which to start. It is perhaps better to only take jobs that have potential. A PVFS patient cannot "try and see" everything. The nature of the illness is such that a patient needs to use foresight, and consider all the implications of a decision.

VOLUNTARY WORK

Where patients are unable to find a suitable part-time/full-time job, they should consider voluntary work. **After a long illness, a patient's confidence is greatly reduced.** The simple routine of an every day job: getting up early, finding transport, speaking to people, being sociable, working, eating and returning home can appear to be an impossible obstacle course.

Fortunately, confidence usually quickly returns. The best jobs are those in which hours are flexible; there is little stress on the patient; the work is not physically demanding; and the patient has some control of the working conditions. **These requirements are easily fulfilled in much voluntary work.** Obviously, a patient may need to choose a suitable job, but there is usually an acceptable selection. If the patient starts with a few hours work per week, it can be quite dramatic how confidence is greatly increased. **With greater confidence, there is less anxiety and stress.** A cycle of benefits accrue to the patient, and enjoyment in life can reach a new high.

CHANGE OF JOB

A change of a job is a feature of life today. Retraining and job mobility are not only part of the political climate, they are a result of developments in industry. When a person changes a job, it may be either because his old job has disappeared, or that he has decided that the new job is better. The latter can be associated with great contentment. PVFS patients have to try to see a change of job in a wider context: that many in the community are being forced to do so (albeit not usually for health reasons), and that they should change to a better job (a job that they can cope with is a better job!).

Nevertheless, a change of job is a major life event and is associated with great stress. It is not a decision that should be undertaken as a result of anger, or a fit of pique. Many patients loved their job before they became ill. These jobs were often difficult and demanding ones which required great energy. **With illness, patients struggle to cope, and one of the first results can be volatile emotions.** Easy irritability can result in sudden outbursts of anger, frustration and tears.

Before a change in job is contemplated it is worthwhile to properly assess the situation and its implications. Ask: was I happy in the job before the illness? If the answer is yes, then consider if the recommendations at the start of this chapter have been given a chance to work. If not, then do so. If yes, consider part-time work. **For patients unhappy in their work before their illness, their illness can be a good opportunity to change jobs.** However, it is still important to consider what is wanted from life, what makes happiness, and what is attainable. **One must be able to**

cope easily with a new job. It is unwise at this stage to have a job that is too demanding.

A change of job is very stressful because of the different environment. Patients need to establish a rapport with their new colleagues to gain goodwill. In previous jobs, patients may have been highly regarded and thus they might have received understanding. Similarly, there is little information on the new environment: Where is the toilet? How does the telephone system work? When is the tea break? Where is the canteen? Where are the envelopes kept? How far is it to the wages department? The list of information can be large. **Patients have to ask for each bit of information and often feel guilty about having to disturb others.** For these reasons, a change of job has to be considered very carefully.

SOCIAL SECURITY BENEFITS

Accepting social security benefits is still something which many patients find difficult. There is the "stigma" attached to not working, perhaps made worse by the individual's own attitudes before the illness. Again, the lack of visible evidence of disability can make others think that the patient is work-shy or malingering. This is yet another time when patients need to realise that they are ill, accept the consequences, and ignore those who do not understand.

Those accepting benefits and help often feel persecuted. Stories in newspapers revealing "scroungers" do not help; instead, they contribute to a general feeling that "handouts" must only go to those in need. The logic is that if there is a system with frequent checks, only those in real need will stand up to these investigations. The logic is flawed. Many of the needy, and some with PVFS, do not have the physical and mental resources to stand up to these checks.

A patient may be more exhausted by getting a benefit than not getting it. For example, a patient receiving invalidity benefit will periodically be summoned to attend a medical assessment. Occasionally, at such a medical, the medical officer may decide that the patient is capable of work. This decision can be a great shock to patients, and even convince them that society is against them. **This is not so, it is the system that is at fault.**

Many patients have struggled up many flights of stairs to attend a medical examination. To the patients this was essential as they needed to attend, and often they were reknown for their reliability before illness. Sadly, their arrival at the examination was their downfall. The medical officer would simply say: I"If you got up the flights of stairs to attend, you cannot be ill". The fact that the patient may be in bed for weeks after this event is of little consequence to the system. **When dealing with the system, patients should not do what they cannot normally do.** If patients had not climbed the stairs, they probably would have got their benefits.

The system, because of society's attitudes, works on frequent checks, double-checks, appeals and adjudications. A recommendation of being incapable of work is only the first step. Immediately, the patient's general practitioner can issue a new sick note, and the whole procedure of reassessment will be started. A patient's doctor is his greatest ally. The system is generally fair and usually works well, but occasionally it does not. Understanding the system and playing the game is the secret. Self-help groups are invaluable in this maze of rules and regulations:

a) **M.E. Association**
4 Corringham Road
Stanford-le-Hope
Essex. SS17 0AH
Tel (01375) 642466 Fax (01375) 360256

b) **Action for M.E.**
PO Box 1302
Wells
Somerset. BA5 1YE
Tel (01749) 670799 Fax (01749) 672561

c) **Westcare**
155 Whiteladies Road
Clifton
Bristol
BS8 2RF
Tel (0117) 923 9341 Fax (0117) 923 9347

There are a great many benefits available:

a) severe disablement allowance
b) disability living allowance (care and mobility)
c) invalid care allowance
d) disability working allowance
e) statutory sick pay
f) incapacity benefit
g) family credit
h) housing benefit
i) social fund, cold weather payment, community care grant, etc

The best explanations of the system are in **Dr Charles Shepherd**'s book, "Living with ME", Cedar, 1992; and **Dr Anne Macintyre**'s book "Chronic Fatigue Syndrome: how to live with it", Thorsons, 1998.

CONCLUSION

There is a great temptation to confuse quantity with quality. Having £10.00 to spend does not mean that the purchase would be better than if there was only 10 pence to spend. Obviously, the chances are that it will be better, but if great effort is put into thinking about the situation, then a more appropriate object may be bought for 10 pence.

Some time off, or part-time work may be necessary, however, this should not be regarded as a solution to the patient's problems. **Instead, it is an opportunity to test how much can be done.** Often, with time off, a patient can become so worried and preoccupied with not improving that he does not attempt to see what he can do. Initially, it is best to look upon part-time work as "test periods" rather than "solutions".

PVFS patients should use their brain more than their muscles; it recovers first and it uses less energy. Because of the need to avoid wasted effort, patients have to identify their priorities. **The combination of thinking first, and concentrating on the important areas of life is a winning duo.**

SUMMARY

1. Employment is an important part of life. It must be valued. Unemployment has many adverse effects, but recovery is more important.

2. To remain employed: stop unnecessary exertion; minimise all walking; think before any action; adopt unwind techniques and increase sleep; and stop all social engagements.

3. Sick leave is not an easy answer. If patients require sick leave, they should plan on at least 3 months, often it is 6-9 months. For recovery, do not substitute other activities for work.

4. Returning to work is a delicate task and requires careful planning and much thought. Ideally, part-time work is recommended with a slow increase in the hours of work, being guided by the patient's diary.

5. Although unemployment is a major life-event, it is an opportunity to consider what has happened. Also ask: What do I want? What will make me happy? What can I get?

6. Part-time work is useful for many patients when they are having difficulties with their job. It is also the recommended route for a return to work. Patients should beware of new part-time jobs, and taking any new job.

7. Voluntary work is frequently the ideal way of returning to the work routine with a minimum of stress and anxiety. Confidence can quickly return.

8. A change of job can be a good or bad decision. Consider carefully the implications. Take a job in which it is easy to cope.

9. Social security benefits are complicated. Know the system and what is being expected of you. Get advice early and do not be naive.

10.Use sick leave or unemployment as an opportunity to identify the priority areas of life. Determine how you have arrived at your current situation. Start thinking of what should be done before rather than after the event.

CHAPTER TWELVE
YOUNG PEOPLE

The "Little People" have always had a fascination for children. In the famous incident of the Cottingley fairy photographs, two young girls claimed to have photographed fairies in July 1917. It later transpired that the girls had used cut-out figures to fake the photographs. However, what is more interesting is that the girls admitted to faking the photographs but still insisted that they had seen the fairies. The reason that they faked the photographs was that adults did not believe their stories.

One can understand children having a vivid imagination, but when an adult recounts a childhood experience it should perhaps be given further consideration. Thus, should the story by Mrs G Herbert in 1928 that she saw a "little wizened man eighteen inches high with a little pointed hat, slightly curved at the front, a doublet and little short knicker things," be dismissed? Often the children are not alone when they have witnessed the presence of the Little People. In 1929 a five year-old girl and her eight year-old brother saw a tiny pilot in a plane with a wing-span of 15 inches fly over their garden fence. Whilst 3 girls in Kilkhampton saw a "little man in a tiny red car driving around in circles". More recently, in 1979 four children (aged 8-10 years) saw about 60 people riding around in little red and white cars.

For PVFS patients, it is important to note a number of characteristics of the Little People. First of all, these accounts show that the Little People are usually driving around, often with mechanised transport. Secondly, the descriptions mention that the Little People were "very happy looking", and that in their presence the children were "awfully happy". I feel that PVFS patients can greatly benefit from looking at their illness as an invasion of the Little People. **The illness will have catastrophic effects on their lives, but there is also the possibility of much happiness.**

For young people, there are also great lessons. The smaller you are, there is the perception that you are happier. I believe that this is true. However, I do not think that size is the major factor, but rather that **young people take every opportunity to be happy. How commendable!** Unfortunately, there is a down-side. Sometimes adults feel that young people should be happy always – even when they are ill. This is wrong.

It is important to recognise the special needs of young people. This has been superbly done by **Jane Colby**, a former headmistress, in her book "ME. The New Plague" First and Best in Education, 1996 (ISBN 1-8608-3215-6). Action for ME have helped to form **TYMES** (The Young ME Sufferer) which is billed as the first independent organisation for young people. With an energetic coordinator and editor (Anna Grace Lidstone) there is a quarterly newsletter, support services and a website!!

In many ways I find that young people are easier to manage than adults. **This is because the relationship is not as complicated, and the young are easier to**

171

convince of a sensible course of action. My approach with managing young people is as for adults. However there are several areas with a different emphasis, and I shall address these in this chapter as follows: honesty, daily diary, contracts, activities, school, university and the future.

HONESTY

Young people are great realists. They see things as they are and are not as conditioned as adults. Initially, they do not pretend and face reality. Therefore, **adults should not try and protect young people, but be honest and truthful.** Then, a good strategy can be worked out and better recovery from illness guaranteed. If one is honest, even with children as young as 6 years, a helpful relationship can develop. This should not be surprising as young children throughout time have been able to deal with disasters. It is critical that this approach is taken as recovery depends on the cooperation of the child. **The parent cannot do what is required for the child.** The parent is able to only help. By minimal involvement of the child and lack of total honesty, many recoveries have been delayed.

DAILY DIARY

Many parents want to do the diary for the child. This is wrong. Children as young as 6 years can be taught to do a diary. Sometimes it means that symbols have to be used. However, as with adults, **the patient is the one who**

is required to do the daily diary. This emphasises the importance of the diary, and also brings home to children how they may use the diary for recovery.

All of the chapters on the five steps to better recovery apply to young people. **They need to understand energy.** There is the need for at least 10 hours sleep. There is the need for trying to teach the patient the art of unwinding. Indeed in many cases, young people have found it easier to learn the art of unwinding compared to adults. Energy is gained in the same way as adults.

Energy is more easily lost as a child. Fortunately, this is physical energy, and **children lose mental energy much less than adults.** Children do not have the anger and frustration of adults. They also do not ruminate and dwell on subjects, the way older PVFS patients do. Again, they are not as stressed as adults. Unfortunately, **the emotional energy of relationships can be worse in children.** There can be great attempts to get their own way, with much crying and tantrums. At these times, it is important for parents to be firm and not give in to unreasonable demands. If this occurs, more problems are created than solved now and in the future.

Energy must be made to last. As in adults, **boredom periods are very important.** Over the years, I found that children accept boredom periods more easily than adults. Then, it occurred to me that boredom periods are an integral part of a child's life. How many times are children made to sit or be quiet when it is the opposite of what they want to do? Simply, **children are already conditioned to boredom periods.** So, yet again, for children the steps to better recovery are already a part of their life. **The required change in lifestyle is much less than in an adult.**

CONTRACTS

I like contracts and deals. I have always made them with my children and I make them with patients. It works very well. It works because it is really the "barter" system which was in existence before money. When there are two people, one does something for the other, and the latter returns the favour by doing something else. **The simple system of contracts is loved by children and prepares them for life in the real world.** I have frequently come across the parent who is trying to cheer the child up by buying new presents. Usually, the child is unwell because he has not stayed within his energy levels. The child is then faced with further mental stimulation by the new present. The child is not very enthusiastic about the present as he is too tired. The parent feels hurt and resolves to spend even more money on the next present. **The vicious cycle is repeated, and made worse.**

My approach is to ask children to stay within their energy limits. This will be reflected in the daily diary scores. If they manage to do well over a week, they deserve a reward. **The child should specify the reward and it should not be too expensive**, a special magazine is ideal. If the child's diary scores are not better, the child does not get a reward. **One should not give the reward irrespective of progress.** This is not a game in which what you do does not matter. It is not about just taking part, it is about winning. Rewards are given only to winners.

If a child has had a really bad week, for example with an infection, it is reasonable for there to be a small present. One would do the same with an adult, perhaps with a present such as a small bar of chocolate. However, **I must say that I believe a long cuddle or telling them a funny**

joke is much more helpful. Christmas presents and birthdays are always a great problem area. **Parents often believe that the ill child should get the most expensive present.** This can result in jealousy if there are other children in the family. I believe that the ill child should be subject to the same rules as the rest of the family. After all, in later life, equal treatment of all is supposed to be an objective of society. Therefore I do not believe in buying the child a toy shop (Figure 27). Instead, I believe that a special present could be better received than many expensive ones. **The key is to give children presents that they really want.** How do you know if someone really wants something? My rule is that they should want it for at least 3 months.

Parental income is not an important factor in children's recovery. The most important factor is the time that a parent spends with a child. If parents give freely of their time, there will always be great benefits to children. More importantly, this applies if the children are ill, poor, or healthy.

ACTIVITIES

How young people spend their time is just as important as in adults. Over the last years, the single greatest change in management has been **the need to regulate young people's use of videos, computer games and music.** This approach cannot be emphasised too much. In the past, as these activities did not involve physical exertion, they were deemed to be "rest". This is wrong as there is great mental use of energy. I have seen too many people who spend all day in bed "resting" while watching videos,

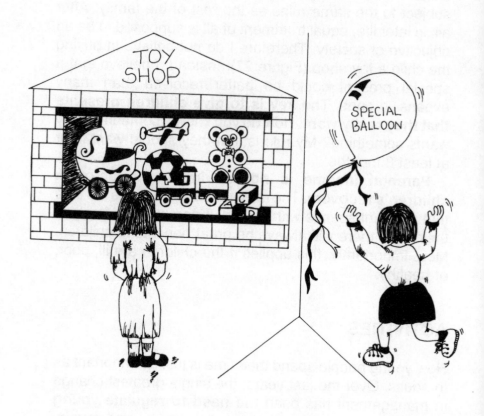

Figure 27 Many or one?
Parents are tempted to give their children a toy shop of new toys. One special toy is better, uses less concentration, is more appreciated and cheaper.

listening to music and playing computer games. **These young people do not recover: the proof of the pudding is in the results.** These activities have to be regulated into half hour periods, and preceded by boredom periods. **There should be no more than one and a half hours of music or a video in any one day.** If scores are under 5/10, there should be no computer games. **These rules have to be explained to young people, and parents must insist on their implementation.** It is like all good parenting and not unlike a young person must be home by 10 o'clock at night.

Visitors are also a great use of energy. I have known young people in bed all day with a continuous stream of their friends visiting them. These patients do not recover. Bed is for lying down with your eyes closed and with no noise in the room. Nothing else will do. Visitors should be regulated to no more than two per day **and** only if there is a better score than the previous average. **Visitors should not stay more than 45 minutes.** This is not a holiday camp, it is about an ill person wanting to get better.

SCHOOL

Most parents have a great worry of young people losing time away from school. This is reasonable but may not help matters. My position is that **all that is learnt up to 11 years at school can be learnt in one good year.** From 11-18 years, in two good years the work can be learnt. Therefore **my objective is to get the young person well rather than worry about lost time at school.** I have seen many parents trying to encourage young people to return to school when they are only 5/10 in their diary scores.

Others have insisted that the school provide home tutors. My approach is for the young person to understand energy and return to school when the diary scores are 8/10. **If this is done there is better progress.** Each time a young person tries to return to school and fails, confidence is destroyed. If young people are able to follow the plan in this book, a return to school should be possible in 10-12 months. Then, all work can be learnt and no time will be lost. **As always, does one focus on a single objective (getting better) or have many** (getting better, going to school, doing well etc)?

The difficulties at school are not only with learning. If this were so, a return to school would not be too difficult. However, school also involves considerable physical activities (walking to classes, stairs etc) and mental activities (explaining the illness to friends, saying no to parties etc). In addition, there are all the other problems of the young, such as peer group pressure, teasing, rivalry, jealousy etc. As with working, if a patient is at school and scoring 5/10, it is easier to remain at school. There should be a good choice of subjects: mathematics needs a lot of concentration; some subjects (eg geography, history) require much memory; english and home economics can be recommended. In some schools, it is possible for the student to do only mornings. **All that is said on the chapter on employment applies to school.** It is equally important that problems are carefully considered.

UNIVERSITY

To go to University is an ambition of most young people. Their parents are proud of them and there is great hope and adventure in their lives. It is therefore a great disaster when someone has to drop out of University because of illness. As with school, there is initial optimism that the long summer holidays will result in recovery. **When this does not happen, there can be great depression.** The first thing to realise is if one had to drop out of University, recovery will take many months. The more usual course is that an individual needs a year to deal with the illness.

The plan as described in this book requires total commitment. There is no time for a social life or attempts to keep up with university work. **A total change of lifestyle is required.** The aim is to get the diary scores back to 8/10. It will take time and an understanding of energy. As many university students are smart, they frequently think that there is an easy way. **The steps in this book are not easy.**

A return to university, as a return to work, must not be underestimated. The course may need to be reconsidered: is it possible to do fewer subjects, especially initially? can the mix of subjects be changed? It is also important to consider the accommodation: is it possible to get into halls of residence? can the bedroom be close to the dining hall? who will be making the meals? **Time must be taken to consider the practical aspects of a return to university life.** If this is not done, the previous mistakes can be easily repeated. Extracurricular activities must be stopped for the first term back. The object is not to let scores fall below 7/10. During the vacation, there should be no holiday jobs unless scores have averaged 8/10. It can be very hard for students. At least if there is no social life, financial spending is greatly reduced. However, **financial concerns must not be considered greater than good health.** Nevertheless, young people at university recover faster

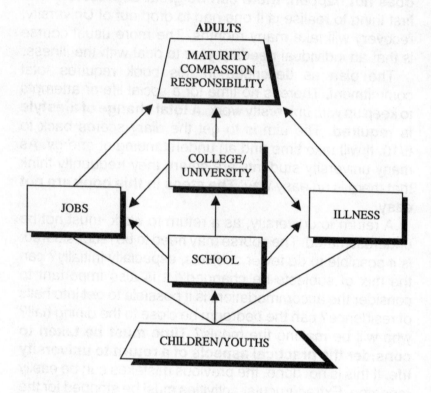

Figure 28   Life
Life involves progress from a child to an adult. There are many ways of learning the requirements of adulthood: responsibility, compassion and maturity. School, College/University are only one route. Working in jobs and illness can also achieve the same result.

180

and more predictably than other adults. **This is especially so if it is possible to focus their intellect on getting better.**

THE FUTURE

It is helpful here to consider how one progresses from a child to an adult (Figure 28). As an adult, it is hoped that one has become mature by accepting personal responsibility and acquiring compassion for others. There are many ways in which this can be achieved. Indeed, one can say that **illness may be a fast track to adulthood.** It is certainly a great teacher to those who want to learn about life.

What is missing in Figure 28 is that one becomes educated and trained at school and university. In the past, university students were guaranteed jobs, but this is no longer true. I meet very many young people who have completed university but still do not know what job they want. I believe that **students should know what job they want before they go to university.** Several PVFS patients have found that once they drop out of university, they recognise that they should not have been there in the first place. This is another example of how illness may ultimately save time and expense.

Almost all PVFS patients who have recovered and returned to school or university were able to quickly catch up. I believe that this was because **illness had focused their thoughts and they were now more committed.** Often in life, we need good reasons to work harder and better. I like the story of how a young boy knows if his face is clean after he has washed it. The answer is that he looks at the towel he has used to dry his face. Many in the population go through school and university without asking if this is what they should do. They have washed their faces and assumed that they are clean. Illness makes them look at the towel to confirm what they are doing.

SUMMARY

1. Adults should not try and protect young people but be truthful and honest. The parent cannot do what is required for the child.

2. Young people have to do the diary themselves, even if it means using symbols.

3. The system of contracts and rewards is easily understood by young people. For presents, quantity and expense cannot replace careful thought in deciding on a special present.

4. Parents need to regulate the use of videos, computer games and music. Visitors use up much energy and must be restricted.

5. Children quickly catch up time lost at school so efforts should be focused on getting children better.

6. Students who drop out of university because of illness need to change their lifestyle.

7. Illness allows young people to become mature by accepting personal responsibility and acquiring compassion for others.

CHAPTER THIRTEEN
ALTERNATIVE MEDICINE

In Cambridge, there once lived a haulage contractor called Thomas Hobson (1544-1631). His company was nationally known and his stables had the largest stock of horses. Mr Hobson cared greatly for his horses. If a horse worked one day, it was given the next day as a rest day. To ensure that his horses were properly looked after, he devised a complicated system of rotation. However, the system worked very simply. When someone wanted to hire a horse, they always got the horse nearest the door. Hobson made such an impact that his name has been incorporated into the English language. "Hobson's choice" is a choice in which one has no alternative.

It is sad that Thomas Hobson should be remembered for how his system worked, rather than for his care of horses. Traditional medicine can sometimes suffer in this way. **It can be forgotten that the system in which traditional medicine operates was designed to protect the patient from charlatans and quacks.** I use "traditional medicine" to reflect medicine as approved by the General Medical Council and taught in medical schools in the West.

I receive new treatments for PVFS patients every few

183

weeks. Nearly all of these treatments are not tested and will benefit less than 0-5% of patients; they cannot be recommended. The more popular alternative treatments are discussed in this chapter under the following general groups:

Group	Results
Historic treatments	Good
Unwind techniques	Good
Food medicine	Poor
Detoxification	Poor
Recent treatments	Variable

The treatments that I shall discuss are not all the treatments available, but the ones that are most offered to patients. My general groups are also my personal interpretation of the main actions of the treatment. My personal perceptions of the usefulness of these remedies are also stated. **Some of these treatments have been tried on many patients and may have a place in patient management.** However, I do not believe that their role should be major, but rather to augment the understanding of energy.

Alternative medicine often has success rates of 0-30%; whereas in modern medicine with agents such as antibiotics, the success rate can be more than 90%. **A lower success rate can mean that a patient may never find success.** In addition, many treatments improve rather than cure patients.

Whenever there have been groups of people, there has always been a need to have an alternative. The alternatives that I shall discuss in this chapter have been selected. They are treatments which offer a different approach to the patient's problems, and which some have found helpful. This is an area of "fringe" medicine. **There are few objective comparisons of the treatment with established medical practice.**

Many are outside the National Health Service and so patients have to pay. **It is believed that patients who pay are more appreciative.** Unfortunately, some treatments can be very expensive. There are sad stories of PVFS patients who have taken out second mortgages on their homes to pay for treatment. Some patients have been made bankrupt. **Patients should not have unrealistic expectations of treatment.** It is totally understandable that patients want to get better, but paying for treatment does not guarantee recovery. **Patients should not pay what they cannot afford.**

HISTORIC TREATMENTS

There is the misconception that alternative medicine is new. In fact, an alternative practice such as acupuncture has been in existence for 2000 years. **Thus, much of traditional medicine is comparatively new.** Perhaps because of its long history, alternative medicine practices are better at explaining illness to the lay public: "imbalance of energy", "presence of toxins", "natural remedies" etc. **The public appreciates the time which alternative medical practitioners take to explain their treatment.** This can be quite refreshing compared to the more paternalistic attitudes of traditional medicine.

Homeopathy
This is derived from two Greek words, "homois" and "pathos", meaning "similar" and "suffering". A homeopathic

185

remedy is one that is able to produce symptoms in a healthy person which are similar to those in the patient. **The treatment causes a stimulation of body defences in patients, and these bring about a recovery.** Much of the initial concepts and knowledge of homeopathy were recorded by a German doctor, called Samuel Hahnemann (1755-1843). Homeopathic treatment is available within the National Health Service and there is a Faculty of Homeopathy, recognised by an Act of Parliament.

Dr Hahnemann was an exceptional man. His intelligence and application at school was such that his teachers did not charge him any fees. When he left school, he spoke eight languages. At the time, many of the medical treatments (e.g. prolonged bleeding of patients, the use of leeches) did much harm. **Dr Hahnemann was very vocal in his opposition to many of these practices.** This was very brave and demonstrates that he was a clear thinker with firm principles.

He concentrated more on studying the patient, and on detailed scientific observation. **He developed three separate approaches to treating an illness:**

a) identify and remove the cause (e.g. poor hygiene).
b) the use of "opposites" **(allopathy)** such as purgatives for constipation. These remedies were not so useful in chronic illnesses, and were best where there was a single symptom. These are of limited value in PVFS.
c) the use of similar remedies **(homeopathy).**

The method of preparation of homeopathic medicine is important. It allows the enhancement of the active component in the medicine, even though it is being diluted. Because there is no apparent dilution effect, the word "potency" is used. Preparations are diluted at least 1:10. At 24 times dilution, there should be no molecules of the original substance, yet these "potencies" have an effect. There is no explanation of this observation.

When a PVFS patient visits a homeopathic doctor, he will be impressed by the time that the doctor spends with him. **A detailed understanding of the patient is a prerequisite of a homeopathic consultation.** Questions will be asked of the family history, the present complaint and the patient's reaction to his complaint. Further, there will be enquiries on food likes and dislikes; menstrual periods; and the emotional state. The doctor will be trying, with this information, to categorise the patient and decide on the best remedy.

Many of the principles of homeopathy are acceptable and used in traditional medicine. It is a safe, cheap and sometimes successful treatment. So, why has homeopathy been regarded as "fringe" medicine?

Part of the answer is in Dr Hahnemann's relationship with other medical colleagues. He attacked **all** of the established medical practices. In the law courts, he lost. When Dr Hahnemann was eighty years old, he decided to run his own homeopathic hospital, it subsequently closed. Another part of the answer is in the changes in medicine. The discoveries of Pasteur and Lister on the treatment of infections allowed a different approach. **Illnesses could be treated by killing the causative organisms. There was little place for Dr Hahnemann's treatment of the whole person.**

I believe that homeopathy has an important role in the management of some problems. Homeopathy was effective and flourished when there were many infectious diseases, and when there was no specific treatment. The situation may not be dissimilar to that with PVFS. Some PVFS patients have had considerable relief of symptoms with homeopathic remedies. **Any approach to treatment that has lasted nearly 200 years cannot be lightly dismissed.** I believe that homeopathy can offer support to some, but not all, patients. It is an alternative for symptomatic relief. It can be adopted as an adjunct to the steps to better recovery that I have advocated in this book.

Acupuncture

Acupuncture has been in existence for over 2,000 years. Chinese medicine sees all the world as a balance between two, opposing forces (Yin and Yang). Taoism ("the way") is the means by which there is harmony between man and these forces. **Illness is a result of disharmony.** Thus, patients often saw their doctor when they were well, and paid the doctor to keep them in harmony. This was preventative medicine at its best, and if individuals became ill, the doctor was not paid. This is quite a different attitude to that in the West.

Centuries of observation have established the acupuncture channels throughout the body. Vital energy flows through these channels. **Thus, if an organ is malfunctioning, there is a deranged flow of energy in a particular channel.** This could be corrected by acupuncture needles placed at appropriate points in the channel. One important consideration is that these points have been determined empirically (as a result of experiments); thus, they work, but no one knows exactly how and why they work.

The success of acupuncture in a patient depends on the skill of the acupuncturist and the complaint. In those that respond, there is usually progressive improvement and only 3-4 treatments are necessary. Best results are in those who have a benefit after the first treatment. Occasionally, there may be late improvements, 3-4 weeks after a course of treatment. **Acupuncture is most effective in pain relief.** The way acupuncture acts is unknown; it may release natural mediators (e.g. endorphins which are natural opiates).

It is a very safe procedure provided that the needles are properly sterilised (to prevent transmission of hepatitis B and C viruses and the HIV/AIDS virus). The usefulness in PVFS is unknown. Most benefit may be in those with pain and breathing difficulties.

Spiritual (Psychic) Healing

The healing of one person by another, by a technique unknown to modern medicine, is usually part of a ritual such as "laying-on of hands". **Some healers activate the patient's own energy, whilst other healers transmit their own (or their God's) energy to the patient.** There are numerous, well-documented reports in religious and medical texts. It is not often successful. When it works, it cannot be explained (i.e. a miracle). It is in the realm of faith, belief and religious conviction.

Among Christians, healing or the restoration of health is often depicted as a manifestation of God's compassion and power. In the four Gospels, well over 20 stories of healings of the sick occur. Immediate cure was bestowed on cases where recovery appeared unlikely. It is not surprising, therefore, that many are attracted to spiritual healing.

Many of my patients have followed the recovery path as in Figure 29. **Despite doing all the right things,**

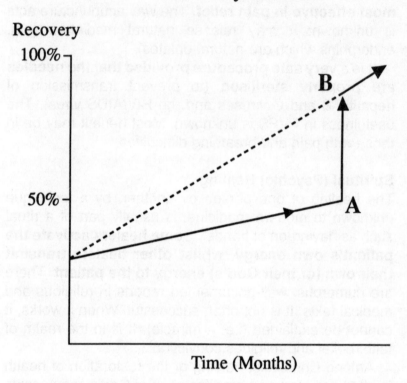

Recovery with Time

Figure 29 Recovery with Time
Many times I have seen patients do all the right things but only have poor recovery (A). I would have expected better recovery (B). At A, something happens (such as laying-on of hands) and there is recovery to B.

patients appear to have poor recovery. Then, something happens and this is especially the case with spiritual healing, and the patient suddenly recovers to what was expected. There are two important observations: recovery is never better than would be expected; and future progress is along the predicted line of recovery. **Could a patient's belief somehow unlock their progress?**

UNWIND TECHNIQUES

Patients gain energy through sleep and unwind techniques (Chapter Eight). **All patients benefit from adopting an unwind technique.** My particular favourite (EMBME) is described in my book ("Unwind" 1991, Dodona Books). **In addition, in "Unwind", Eastern techniques (meditation, Buddhism, Taoism, Zen and Yoga) are described.** The place of Western techniques (Christianity, Psychotherapy, Auto-suggestion, Hypnotherapy, Biofeedback and Visualisation) is also explained. Unwind techniques are very highly recommended.

The difficulty for most patients is that unwind techniques take time to learn; benefits are not felt for 2-3 months. **During this period, patients need to commit themselves to learning a new skill.** Sadly, many patients who have been ill for years are not prepared to learn; they expect to be cured instantly.

Meditation
Meditation is a component of many Eastern techniques and can include a wide range of activities. One definition is **"a family of techniques which have in common a**

191

conscious attempt to focus attention in a non-analytical way and an attempt not to dwell on ruminating discursive thought". (American Journal of Psychiatry, 1982; 139: 267-74). Unwind techniques, aided by controlled breathing and quiet chanting, are common to most forms of meditation. **The object is to get out of the "fight or flight" (ie stress) reaction of modern living.** Apart from the mental peace of such a procedure, there appears to be reduced sympathetic nervous response. Blood pressure, muscle tone and skin conductance also may be lowered. Thus, the whole process is high quality rest; the muscles and the mind are given the right environment for repair of damaged tissues. It is not surprising that all patients can benefit from meditation.

Massage

Touching is a necessary activity for a normal healthy life. **Massage is the ancient art of healing by touch.** Very many ancient Chinese, Indian and Egyptian practitioners have described their art in great detail. In the West, the Swede (Per Henrick Ling) has been responsible for the development of massage techniques. There are several important components.

i)   effleurage (stroking with the whole hand): this is the basic stroke of massage.
ii) péttrisage (kneading, squeezing, rolling): this is very good for improving circulation and removing toxins from affected muscle groups.
iii) friction (deep circulatory movements with thumbs): this can be painful and should be used on muscle groups, especially when there is tension.
iv) tapotement (hacking or chopping of muscles): this

improves circulation or affected muscles and is often combined with (ii).

Massage is a complicated subject and patients who are interested should get more information from books on the subject. **Acupressure** and **Shiatsu** (finger pressure) are like acupuncture without needles. One presses with the thumb over specific points for 20 seconds, releases and waits for 10 seconds, and then repeats up to 5 times. Pressure on the inside of the left wrist is useful for nausea. Pressure on the middle of the upper lip helps pain. Pressure on the lobe of the left ear helps sleep.

Aromatherapy uses essential oils (aromatic chemicals) and is often combined with massage. The **Alexander technique** focuses on postural improvement to cure or prevent many disorders. **Reflexology** is an ancient Chinese and Egyptian technique which unblocks energy channels throughout the body.

T'ai Chi Chuan
Usually known as T'ai Chi, this has become very popular. This ancient Chinese technique applies Taoist principles to the art of movement. The principles of balance between the opposing forces of **Yin** (dark, feminine, passive) and **Yang** (light, male, active). Yin represents the interior of the body and solid organs, whereas Yang represents the exterior of the body and hollow organs. **T'ai** is the Chinese word meaning a centre point which is the dividing line between Yin and Yang. **Chi** is the energy force of life. The Taoists believed that if you can release and direct the energy force within the body, by a series of exercises, the balance in the body is regained and so stress and illness can be removed.

Self-hypnosis

In hypnosis, a trance-like state is induced in which the mind accepts suggestions. There is total mental concentration but physical relaxation. **Hypnotism is not a treatment in itself,** although because it is advertised as a "cure" for smoking and obesity, it is perceived by the public as such. It is important to recognise that hypnosis is the acceptance of suggestion. It can be very useful in dealing with stress and increasing an individual's ability to unwind.

FOOD MEDICINE

Food is an important factor in recovery from PVFS. There is no doubt that some patients on bizarre diets (ice-cream and chips, cauliflower and sugar etc) may develop nutritional deficiencies. However, for patients who have a normal diet and are eating within a family, such nutritional deficiencies are rare. Indeed, the most common complaint is that patients are putting on weight as they have reduced their activity. **For these patients, no special foods are required. However, there are some frequent and popular food medicines:**

Herbalism
The use of plants in healing probably dates from man's earliest existence. Fresh rather than frozen vegetables are advised. There are many "decoctions" (prepared by boiling) which can be used for many of the complaints of PVFS patients. Certainly, many modern medicines have been derived from plants, however in PVFS it has been difficult to assess herbal remedies.

Folk Medicine

Chronic fatigue is considered in a book entitled "Folk Medicine" by Dr D C Jarvis, Pan Books Ltd, 1961. This recommends the use of honey, apple-cider vinegar, baked beans and sea food. A few patients may be helped, but perhaps the most important quote in the book (for patients with PVFS) is that of the former president of Dartmouth College: **"I never run if I can walk; I never stand if I can sit; I never sit if I can lie down."**

Royal Jelly

Royal Jelly is the food for the Queen Bee. **It is special and for centuries it has been used to treat a variety of ailments.** Unfortunately, there are two major drawbacks. The effects are not predictable; and it can be difficult to obtain Royal Jelly. Some patients benefit from the fact that Royal Jelly can relax them and help sleep. Others claim a reduction in muscle pain and the ability to think more clearly. Some manufacturers have been selling "ordinary" honey as "Royal Jelly". One patient ate three different preparations of Royal Jelly to be sure that he was getting the real thing. I would rather patients to have a greater emphasis on understanding energy.

Probiotics

Probiotics are bacteria which are "friendly" and can replace more harmful bacteria in the colon. These bacteria are concentrated in capsules which can be taken in between meals. **The bacteria then multiply in the colon and displace other more harmful agents such as candida.** Some of these bacteria eg **Lactobacillus acidophilus**, are also found in live yoghurt. They are killed in pasteurised yoghurt and so are of no use. Yoghurt is also a very easily digested food and can be recommended for PVFS patients. However, the role of probiotic capsules or powder is unproven.

DETOXIFICATION

Dental Amalgam Removal
Mercury is present in **dental amalgam** which is used for filling teeth. **In individuals with very many fillings, it has been suggested that removal of these fillings can be associated with a great improvement.** Unfortunately, removal of all fillings cannot be done on the National Health Service and may cost several thousand pounds. In addition, removal of the amalgam causes a large amount of mercury to be released; and such dental procedures may result in a patient having a relapse. It is very unlikely that many patients will benefit from amalgam removal, and I would not recommend it.

Colonic Lavage
During the early 1990's, these treatments were very popular. **The reasoning is that the large colon becomes overloaded with toxins and the patient requires repeated enemas to remove these toxins.** Alternative names for this treatment are colonic irrigation or colonic lavage. A colonic therapist will insert a large volume of warm water though the anus into the large bowel, removal of the water is accompanied by faeces and toxins. A therapist can charge £50.00 per visit and this treatment can be expensive. It cannot be recommended.

RECENT TREATMENTS

These treatments have recently become popular in the West although they have a long tradition in the East. As these treatments have been extensively advertised in magazines and newspapers, I receive many letters and telephone calls on their usefulness. My comments here are brief and interested patients should get more detailed information. However many patients are happy with the following details:

Trancutaneous Electrical Nerve (TEN) Transmission
This treatment involves the placing of surface pads (electrodes) on the skin, and passing a current through them. The technique is most helpful in the control of pain, but is probably not as successful as acupuncture. Interestingly, the Romans used electric eels in a similar way to control pain.

Sound Waves
Ultrasonic machines which produce vibrations of variable frequency can be bought. The principle of the technique is that healthy cells vibrate at a particular frequency which may become abnormal with disease. The machine allows the affected cells to return to their original frequency. This treatment is probably best in the control of pain.

Colour Therapy
Although colour therapy has been used by ancient Egyptians and Indians, it has only recently become fashionable in the West. The principle is that each colour vibrates at a different rate and can be used to return diseased cells to their correct vibration, as with sound

waves. The Egyptians used coloured rooms for healing, and one does not necessarily need to see the colour as blind people can benefit. **Crystals** and **gems** have been claimed to work in the same way as colours. The healing forces of gems and crystals are reflected by their colour. Crystals are particularly effective in unwinding and relieving stress.

CONCLUSION

One criticism of modern medicine is that it is too specialised. Doctors become experts on a particular part of the body or particular illnesses. **They appear to know more and more about less and less.** Some feel that this approach has resulted in doctors being narrow-minded, even short-sighted. **The techniques mentioned in this chapter are different. They consider the whole person, not just a symptom or a part of the body.** They are also of another time; most have existed for hundreds of years. In the past, specific drug therapy was not available, and there were also many infectious diseases. Successful treatment depended on understanding the whole person and using all of the body's resources to fight the illness. This situation may have many similarities with that of a PVFS patient.

What should a patient do? The answer depends on the patient and the patient's dilemma is illustrated in Figure 30. Throughout this book, I have suggested that patients should become responsible for their own health. In time, they will know more about their illness in relation to their bodies than their doctor. Similarly, as alternative medical techniques have not been fully tested (or accepted) by the

CHOOSE !!

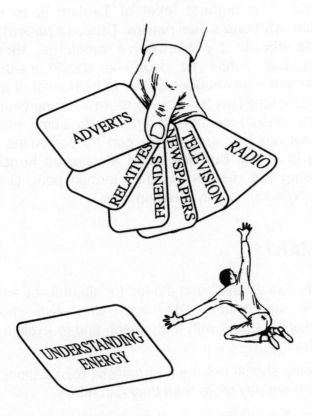

Figure 30   Choose!!
Patients are bombarded by information from adverts, relatives, friends, newspapers, television and radio. There is too much choice; there are too many cures. I believe that the most important card is not usually in the pack to choose from. The most important card, as explained in this book, is an understanding of energy. Although not as attractive as others, it is likely to be more successful.

199

medical profession, patients may easily acquire more information than their doctor.

In films of the old Wild West, there is the common situation where the hero says: "A man must do what a man must do". **The highest level of Taoism is to be in harmony with one's own nature. Thus, if a patient feels that he should try alternative medicine, then he should.** But, before he does, he should make one commitment – he should promise to be honest. If after a reasonable time (say 3-4 weeks); there is no improvement, then, he should be honest enough to admit that the treatment has not worked. He can try something else. **Trying is living, but one must always be honest in assessing the results.** As the German poet, Goethe, states: "Wisdom is only found in truth."

SUMMARY

1. There has always been a need for alternatives and the public appreciates the time alternative medical practitioners take with the patient, and to explain their treatment.

2. Patients should not have unrealistic expectations and should not pay more than they can afford.

3. Alternative medicine is often "older" than traditional medicine, but the success rates are 0-30% as compared to more than 90% in traditional medicine.

4. Historic treatments (homeopathy, acupuncture and spiritual healing) usually have good results.

5. Unwind techniques (meditation, massage, T'ai Chi and self-hypnosis) also usually have good results.

6. Food medicine (herbalism, folk medicine, Royal Jelly and probiotics) usually have poor results.

7. Detoxification techniques (dental amalgam removal, colonic lavage) also have poor results.

8. Recent treatments (TEN, sound waves, and colour therapy) are based on older techniques that have recently become fashionable, but have variable results.

9. Patients need to choose if they should try a particular technique. There are more techniques than patients, but I feel understanding energy is the most difficult and the most successful.

CHAPTER FOURTEEN
MANAGEMENT

Sir Edward Halse, physician to King George III, was amazed at the success of a quack doctor called Dr Rock. When these two gentlemen first met, he could not resist asking:

"How can you, without any education, skill or knowledge of medicine live in such style with a town house, country house and carriage? Whereas I, allowed to possess some knowledge have none of these things."

Rock, slightly amused, replied: "How many people have passed since you asked your question?"

"About a hundred" answered the doctor.

"And how many out of that hundred think you possess common sense?"

"Possibly one" replied Sir Edward.

"Then", said Rock "That one comes to you, and I take care of the other ninety-nine."

PVFS patients are less than one in a hundred, nevertheless, **it is equally important for these patients to be discerning.** There are many who feel able to give advice, and indeed the problem for PVFS patients is that they are often given too much advice. Yet, patients need help. Ideally, their doctor should be aware of their illness, its natural history and the value of supportive treatment. **Equally, patients should understand their affliction and have realistic expectations of their doctors and themselves.**

In the last decade, medical management of PVFS has dramatically changed. These changes mean that there are now acceptable models of patient management. In this chapter, medical management will be considered as follows: medical knowledge, doctor's role (medical assessment and treatment) and the patient's role.

MEDICAL KNOWLEDGE

Despite advances in medical knowledge of PVFS, it is still in its infancy. This is not because the syndrome is new. Indeed, there are extensive descriptions of the disorder, probably at least as early as the seventeenth century (Chapter Two). However, it is only recently that there has been a greater understanding of PVFS. This change has been due to a combination of social circumstances and medical education. **In the past, medical students were taught that recovery from viral illnesses always occurs within weeks.** If the patient did not recover, it was because of "low moral fibre" or even "malingering". As with many other dogmas, this was wrong. PVFS is one exception to quick recovery from viral illness.

Social circumstances have also changed in the last decade. **In particular, individuals have much greater expectation of the medical profession and society spends more time and effort on being well.** These latter two factors have combined to motivate patients with PVFS to keep seeing their doctor. Much of the recent research into PVFS has been prompted by patients insisting that they are ill, and eventually well-motivated doctors finding evidence to support patients' claims. In some cases, the doctors themselves have been ill and faced with scepticism, they have instigated their own research. **Thus, a combination of factors has contrived to increase research and interest in PVFS.** In retrospect, it is not surprising that an illness which produces such morbidity should eventually force itself to the attention of the medical profession.

Current medical knowledge allows some definite statements to be made about PVFS. The most important is that the disease exists. To most sufferers, this may appear to be an obvious statement. Yet, until recently many medical practitioners did not accept the existence of the illness. For medical progress to be made, the first major step is the general acceptance of the disease entity. Only then can there be widespread cooperation, observation, research and funding into the condition. This stage has been reached and now there is every likelihood of major breakthroughs in our understanding of PVFS. Doctors who qualified three decades ago did not study PVFS at medical school. This has changed. **Doctors at medical school are now taught the existence of PVFS.**

A critical question is what causes the disease. The answer to this question is not easy and there is likely to be a number of factors. At the moment, it appears that the most important mechanism is immunological. The attempt by the body to deal with the initial infection results in serious damage to the immune system. Cells and organs throughout the body are caught up in the process. **It is comparable to a civil war in which innocent**

bystanders become involved, and the effects of the war influence subsequent generations.

Thus, in some patients there is widespread damage to the body during the initial assault, and this damage takes years to repair. In other patients, there may not be such widespread damage, but instead the immune system is decimated. This is comparable to the state of an army after a major war. It is unable to effectively deal with other aggressors. **For these patients, the major problem is dealing with subsequent infection which may not only last longer, but also deplete the available resources further.**

What does this information mean for the patient and the doctor? To continue my analogy of a war further, the implication is that the body slowly recovers. However, in a very small number, the onslaught may have been too much, and after a variable period of maladjustment, a more serious illness may develop. Such casualties are rare. For the majority there has to be a slow adjustment to changed circumstances. **If one is injured, there is little value in spending too much time in the consideration of why one became injured.** A more productive position is one that rationalises the injury and adopts a lifestyle to accommodate the new circumstances.

In this book, I am advocating a pragmatic approach. The body has been dealt a potentially mortal blow. It makes sense to change one's lifestyle so that the demands are reduced, thereby allowing the body to recover. In the future, there will be methods that will allow manipulation of the immune system. **Such methods will greatly improve the outlook of patients with PVFS.** In the past few years, cognitive behaviour therapy and graded exercise programmes have been suggested for PVFS patients.

Cognitive Behaviour Therapy (CBT)

In 1990, a model for PVFS (ME) was proposed in which the authors suggested that patients by avoiding exercise perpetuated their illness, and the answer was appropriate CBT (Journal of the Royal College of General Practitioners 1989; 39: 26-29). My article in response to this paper showed that their model was applicable to only the long-term ill patient. The recently-ill patient often tried to exercise to fitness, and it was the inability to recover which made the long-term ill reduce their exercise. (Ho-Yen DO. British Journal of General Practice, 1990; 37-39). More recently, other workers have claimed that CBT aided recovery by **reducing** patients' belief that their illness was mainly physical, caused by a virus and exercise should be avoided (British Medical Journal, 1996; 312: 22-6). My response to this work was that I achieved similar benefits by **increasing** patients' beliefs in these areas (Ho-Yen DO. British Medical Journal 1996; 312: 1097-1098). So, what is the explanation of these opposing views?

I believe the answer is in CBT. The best of CBT is when there is a collaborative rather than an adversarial approach between doctor and patient; problems are solved; there is education of the patient; sessions are structured; and treatment is time-limited. **Therefore, my approach to management uses the best of CBT.** The difference between my management and those of others is that they insist on "graded exercise", whereas **I do not recommend increasing exercise until diary scores are 8/10.**

Graded Exercise

This usually means a gradual increase in exercise. To the public, there is a vision of someone in a jogging suit running for many hours. However, to those who suggest graded exercise, it may mean someone who was previously in bed all day getting up and walking across the room. In some studies, supervised "graded exercise" amounted to 5-15 mins per week for 12 weeks.

My approach is that patients have a limited amount of energy (money), and they must decide how to spend it. If some want to walk or run, it is up to them, however **they must remain within their energy limits.** My approach changes when patients are able to score 8/10 for at least 4-6 weeks. Then, **exercise should be gradually increased with the objective of patients slowly becoming fit again.**

DOCTOR'S ROLE

Better recovery from PVFS depends on a partnership between the doctor and patient. Like the best partnerships, this will require commitment and responsibility from both. Equally, it should be realised that both are bringing different gifts to the partnership. The doctor's role is in medical assessment and managing treatment.

Medical Assessment
Medical assessment is essential in dealing with any patient. With PVFS patients, it can be more complicated and time-consuming. There are three objectives: to make a diagnosis, be aware of other diagnoses and to identify a patient's problems.

Diagnosis
The diagnosis of PVFS has been discussed in Chapter Four. **It is a clinical diagnosis and there are no specific**

laboratory tests. It is also what is called a "diagnosis of exclusion" (ie other conditions which may produce similar symptoms have to be excluded), and so the diagnosis must be made by a doctor. **In the vast majority of patients, there is no evidence of a continuing viral infection.** In a small number, there is evidence such as IgM antibodies (especially to Coxsackie or Epstein-Barr viruses), or raised IgG antibody titres. Many patients have raised IgG antibody to measles virus, but this is probably a reflection of disturbed immune function rather than continuing infection. It is rare to grow the causative virus in samples from the patient.

Other presumptive evidence that may be found in PVFS are low IgA levels, circulating immune complexes, changes in T (helper), T (suppressor) and natural killer cells. **It must be emphasised that completely normal laboratory results are very common in patients with PVFS.** Although abnormal results can be comforting, both for patient and doctor, they are **not** necessary to make the diagnosis.

Many patients are dismayed at the time taken for doctors to make the diagnosis. This caution of doctors is normal when the diagnosis is one of exclusion. In the past, in one study, the diagnosis was made only when 92% were ill for more than one year, and 39% were ill for more than 11 years. **Matters are now greatly improved and the majority of patients are diagnosed within 6 months (Figure 31).** This study was done a decade ago, but there can still be delay in diagnosis. My impression now is that 80% receive a diagnosis within 6 months, but 5% may be ill for more than 2 years.

Some doctors may have great difficulty in accepting PVFS as the diagnosis. This may be because the patient's

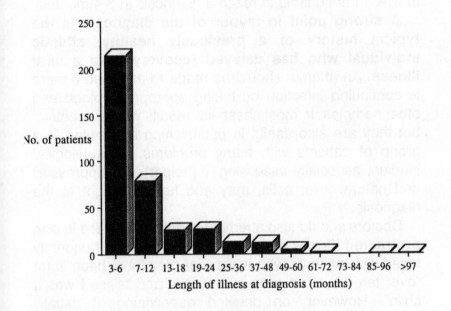

No. of patients

250 —
200 —
150 —
100 —
50 —
0 —

3-6 7-12 13-18 19-24 25-36 37-48 49-60 61-72 73-84 85-96 >97

Length of illness at diagnosis (months)

Figure 31   Length of illness at diagnosis
In one study, diagnosis of the illness has greatly improved. The
majority of patients (56%) were diagnosed when they were ill for 3-6
months, and only 9% were ill for more than 2 years.
(Ho-Yen DO, Scottish Medical Journal, 1988; 33:368–9

history is particularly complicated, possibly with significant emotional problems. Other patients may have obvious psychiatric problems. **It is good practice for a doctor to take time in making a diagnosis.** In some cases, I have said to patients that I am unclear as to the precise diagnosis, but **that in the next 3-4 months, the diagnosis should become obvious.** I have not come across a case in which I am unable to reach a diagnosis in 3-4 months.

A strong point in favour of the diagnosis is the typical history of a previously healthy, athletic individual who has delayed recovery from a viral illness. An attempt should be made to establish if there is continuing infection by taking appropriate blood and other samples. In most cases the results will be negative, but they are also useful in establishing a baseline in a group of patients with many problems. Immunological studies, especially assessing T (helper), T (suppressor) and natural killer cells, may add further weight to the diagnosis.

Doctors should also attempt **to identify if there is one protracted illness or several illnesses.** I am frequently faced with patients who insist that they have been ill for "over ten years" or even "all my life" and "since I was a child". However, on detailed questioning, it usually becomes obvious that the patient behaved normally for much of his life. Usually **it is possible to identify the start of the illness when tiredness was greater than 50% of normal.** The next problem is to determine if there were periods of 6-8 weeks of normality during the years of illness. In most patients, there is not one continuing illness, but two or three attacks of illness. **This is important as patients with second or third attacks do better than patients with a continuing illness.** This is simply because if one can recover once, it is possible to do it again. It is also reassuring to patients and to the doctor.

Other diagnoses
As PVFS is diagnosed by excluding other causes of the patient's complaints, it is particularly important to be aware of other diagnoses. There are several conditions which are frequently confused with PVFS, and which need to be managed differently:

1. Chronic Pain Syndrome:
In this condition, pain of muscles and/or joints is the principal complaint. Patients would often say that they did not mind the tiredness, but the pain was intolerable. Although there is muscle or joint pain in about a third of PVFS patients, the **tiredness is always greater than the pain.** In patients with Chronic Pain Syndrome, the pain may seriously disturb sleep. As with PVFS, reduced sleep makes tiredness worse. Patients should be given pain killers and sleeping tablets to try and improve sleep.

Management of chronic pain syndrome is different from PVFS. Patients are reassured that their pain is not serious, and encouraged to tolerate the pain. **At the end, the pain remains the same but the effect of the pain on the patient is much less.** In contrast with PVFS, the tiredness (and pain) improves with management. Patients should use the daily diary to record scores for pain and tiredness, with hours of sleep.

2. Primary Fibromyalgia Syndrome:
In this condition, there are characteristic tender points in the body (Figure 32). These tender points are different from PVFS in which muscle groups are usually affected,

usually muscles of the limbs. In Primary Fibromyalgia Syndrome, there are tender points over bony areas which does not happen in PVFS. Patients also have a different epidemiology, and I found that the ratio of PVFS to Primary Fibromyalgia Syndrome was 99:1 (British Medical Journal 1994; 309: 1515). **The management of Primary Fibromyalgia Syndrome is to control sleep and increase activities.** This is one condition which benefits from increasing exercise.

Identify Patients' Problems
As with most individuals accustomed to good health, PVFS patients do not adjust well to being ill. Their complaints are many. Their anger and frustration with the medical profession and their situation is intense. Time has to be spent in penetrating this barrier of anger and frustration. Although in all patients the principal complaint is tiredness, in some patients other complaints can be very worrying. Many patients have severe headaches and others can complain of incapacitating dizziness. These complaints have to be treated symptomatically; however, if PVFS is the cause of the complaint, **there is always improvement as the diary scores get better.**

It is essential that there is a good relationship between the doctor and the patient. Both need to be able to trust each other. **Where such trust exists, it is easier for the doctor to identify the patient's problems, ascertain the most likely cause and prescribe the most appropriate treatment.** The important decision as to whether a symptom is due to PVFS, or to something else is for the doctor to make. The doctor will also need to establish if there are other problems, in particular those related to work, finances and relationships. Appropriate

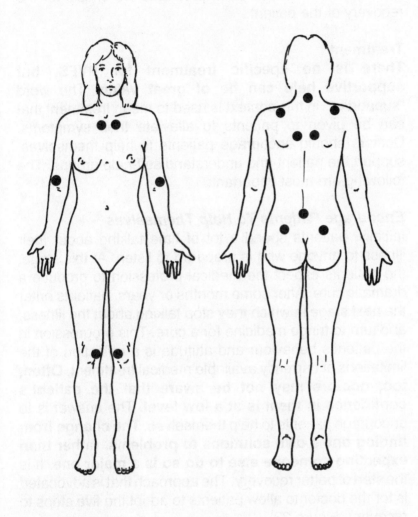

Figure 32   Tender Points
There are tender points at 14 characteristic sites in Primary
Fibromyalgia Syndrome.
(Ho-Yen DO, Physician. 1990: 581–3.)

management of these other problems are critical for the recovery of the patient.

Treatment
There is no specific treatment for PVFS, but supportive help can be of great value. The word "supportive" in this context is used to mean treatment that can be given to patients to alleviate their symptoms. Doctors should encourage patients to help themselves, support the patient and understand self-help groups. The following are most important:

Encourage Patients To Help Themselves
Initially, patients spend a lot of time talking about their illness to anyone who is prepared to listen. At this stage, the patients expect the medical profession to produce a dramatic cure. After some months or years, patients enter the next stage in which they stop talking about the illness, and turn to fringe medicine for a cure. This progression in the patient's behaviour and attitude is a reflection of the limitations of currently available medical treatment. **Often, too, doctors may not be aware that the patient's confidence in them is at a low level.** The answer is to encourage patients to help themselves. **The change from finding one's own solutions to problems, rather than expecting someone else to do so is a major one.** It is the start of better recovery. The approach that is advocated is for the doctor to allow patients to adopt the five steps to recovery (Figure 33).

Support the patient
Perhaps more than anything else, the patient appreciates the doctor's support. Common complaints

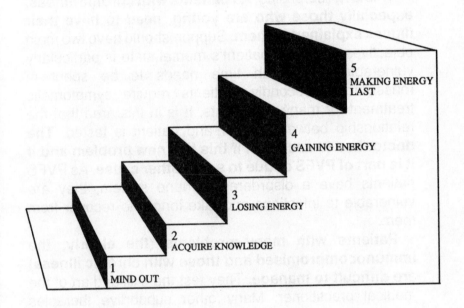

Figure 33 Steps to recovery
There are five main steps to recovery and each step is of varying difficulty. The whole objective is to understand energy. Each step is further explained in separate chapters in this book.

215

are: "My doctor does not believe that I am ill" or "Why does my doctor want me to see a psychiatrist?" These two examples are probably breakdowns in communication rather than lack of support from the doctor. **Nevertheless, they highlight the fact that PVFS patients require a lot of the doctor's time.**

This is not surprising. **All patients with chronic illness, especially those who are young, need to have their illness explained to them.** Support should have two main objectives. First, the patient's mental state is particularly vulnerable and much time needs to be spent in reassurance. Secondly, patients require symptomatic treatment for many complaints. It is in this area that the relationship between doctor and patient is tested. **The doctor has to ascertain if this is a new problem and if it is part of PVFS or due to some other cause.** As PVFS patients have a disordered immune system, they are vulnerable to infections and take longer to recover from them.

Patients with many problems (the elderly, the immunocompromised and those with chronic illness) are difficult to manage. They test the skill and art of the medical practitioner. Many other supportive therapies have been suggested for PVFS. Many of these are considered in the chapter on Alternative Medicine (Chapter Thirteen). Important medical treatments, their effectiveness and disadvantages are:

	Treatment	Success	Problems
1.	Pain killers	Good	Few
2.	Antidepressants	Good	Several
3.	Sleeping tablets	Very good	Several
4.	Anti-fungal measures	Fair	Many

5.	Vitamins and minerals	Poor	Many
6.	Other measures	Poor	Great

As with alternative medicine, some medical practitioners are reluctant to prescribe any of the therapies in the list. The difficulty is that these therapies can have significant disadvantages. Equally, patients can be reluctant to accept medical help. **My position is that the medical profession can offer limited help to PVFS patients, but if the conditions are right such help can be valuable aids.**

1. Pain Killers
If patients moderate their activity, pain is reduced. Pain is also a useful sign; it tells patients that they are doing too much. Patients with muscle pain find it easier to control their activities than patients without muscle pain. A significant number of patients do not have pain but many of these patients may go on to develop muscle pain. I believe that patients should first try to moderate their activities and understand energy. Nevertheless, I recognise that some patients may be helped by medication.

I would initially use **paracetamol**. This is the initial drug of choice. **In about a quarter of patients, sleep is severely disturbed and more potent pain-killers may be required for a short time.** Useful drugs are: **dihydrocodeine (DF-118) Co-codamol, distalgesic or pentazocine (Fortral).** If these are not successful, the non-steroidal anti-inflammatory group of drugs should be considered. **Ibuprofen** is probably the most helpful and Voltarol is worth trying. **For each patient, it is worth trying several pain killers as persistence is frequently rewarded.**

217

2. Antidepressants

My initial management of patients with mild depression is in Chapter Five. **Overall, in about a quarter of patients at some time, antidepressants may be required.** As stated by **Dr David Bell** ("The disease of a thousand names", Pollard Publications, 1991), tricyclic antidepressants can make patients feel like a "zombie", but very small doses of these medications may improve symptoms. The dosage should start at the lowest possible and gradually increase until the patient feels better but does not have a hangover. Three useful agents are **amitriptyline (Tryptizol), doxepin (sinequan) and dothiepin (prothiaden).** Unfortunately, all tricyclic antidepressants have side-effects which may be disturbing. However, if the dose is low, side-effects are minimised and may also settle in 1-2 weeks. Other antidepressants such as **Fluoxetine (prozac), sertraline (lustral), paroxetine (seroxat)** may occasionally be useful. It is worth experimenting. Dr Susan Tainsh of McMaster University has had extensive experience in treating patients and likes **moclobemide (manerix)** for its few side-effects; and particularly recommends **nefazodone (dutonin)** as it is least likely to interfere with sleep architecture.

For PVFS patients, the topic of antidepressants can be very emotive. Patients resist taking antidepressants because of their stigma. **However, tricyclic antidepressants at low dose are good at improving sleep.** Also if you are getting better on antidepressants, you must not suddenly stop taking them. The daily dose needs to be reduced very gradually. Depression can lead to suicide and must be taken seriously. Doctors are happier to prescribe antidepressants rather than sleeping tablets as the former are designed for long term use.

3. Sleeping Tablets

My first approach to patients with sleeping problems is to get them to understand energy. Many patients can be too tired or anxious to sleep and **moderating activity can result in better sleep. At the same time, I recommend unwind exercises.** These may be combined with the traditional remedies of **honey in warm milk, hot drinking chocolate at night or a short massage.** Some patients can also benefit from a long, hot bath; however, other patients may be made considerably worse by a hot bath. If after two months, there is no improvement, sleeping tablets should be considered.

Dr Susan Tainsh of McMaster University uses **clonazepam (rivotril)** for sleep maintenance at a dose of 0.5mg to 2mg two hours before bedtime; and if there is awakening during the night, a further 0.25mg to 0.5mg is given. Dr Tainsh has documented that under 5% of her patients have adverse reactions to this drug, and she has not found that this drug is addictive.

Other drugs, such as **zopiclone (zimovane)** are best for short-term use. It appears to give a good quality sleep and is best initially used as half-dose (3.75mg at bedtime). Although it is less addictive, it can produce a metallic taste in the mouth. Some antidepressants may have a sedative effect, and a few patients have got a better sleep from tricyclic antidepressants, but I do not believe that this was because these patients were depressed. The answer is probably in the pharmacological action of these agents. The intermediate-lasting benzodiazepines are less useful such as **temazepam, lormetazepam and triazolam.** The long-lasting preparations are not recommended. A main drawback of these drugs is that they may become addictive. However, in PVFS patients they should be used for short periods such as 1-3 weeks. **A 3-week course may break a bad sleeping cycle, even though some patients may feel worse whilst on treatment, they are often better when treatment stops.** Generally, it is worth experimenting with several preparations and it is usually possible to find one which benefits the patient.

4. Anti-Fungal Measures

The suggestion that fungal infections such as yeast infection (especially *Candida albicans*) may aggravate PVFS warrants further consideration. Those who are good candidates for yeast infection are women, especially if they are on the contraceptive pill or on an immunosuppressant. In such patients, because of the difficulty in diagnosing low-grade fungal infection, a short course of an anti-fungal drug (eg Nystatin) may be tried. **A few patients have had considerable benefit, but most are unaffected.**

Some practitioners have advocated large doses of nystatin combined with an anti-Candida diet. There are various claims for the success of this approach, but in my experience only a few patients benefit. Diets can be very time consuming and expensive (Chapter Ten), and often the patient has to still recover from PVFS. **It is likely that candida (or other yeasts) infection may make PVFS worse, but that such infection is not the cause of PVFS.** Nevertheless, some patients, especially those with long-lasting illness may have improvement of their abdominal complaints with an anti-Candida diet.

5. Vitamins and Minerals

Extra vitamins, especially large doses of Vitamin C, B6

and B12 have been used in PVFS patients. My feelings about extra vitamins (Chapter Ten) are that **they are unnecessary in an individual who is eating normally.** Recently, it has also been suggested that extra minerals may be of benefit. In particular, weekly injections of **magnesium** have been advocated (Lancet, 1991; 337: 757-760). Low red blood cell magnesium may result from many other conditions such as inactivity (which can be common in PVFS patients) or hypothyroidism. The role of magnesium in PVFS is unproven and most other workers have not confirmed the initial results. It is probably not wise to give magnesium to patients unless they have low red blood cell magnesium and have normal kidney function.

Zinc is an essential mineral for good health. It also has anti-viral effects and is important in immune function, but is present in many foods and supplements are usually not necessary. Similarly, it has been suggested that **selenium** may moderate the individual's immune response to viral infections. However, there is no good evidence that selenium supplements may benefit PVFS patients.

6. Other Measures
As each fortnight goes by, there is a new suggested measure that may benefit PVFS patients. Suggestions may be totally anecdotal, such as bee stings or electric shocks. Alternatively, they may have some scientific basis. For example, **Coenzyme Q10** has been advocated. This enzyme is present in mitochondria (which are the batteries of human cells) and play an important role in energy production. This substance may also neutralise harmful toxins, but there is no study showing benefit of this enzyme to many PVFS patients.

Unlike the position with bacterial infections, specific

treatment with **anti-viral agents** is limited. Thus, there are anti-viral agents against some herpes viruses which are very effective such as **acyclovir (zovirax), ganciclovir (cymevene) and azidothymidine (retrovir).** None of these agents have been shown to have proven benefits for PVFS patients. In the future, anti-viral agents may have a role in specific treatment. There are considerable risks to patients in adopting unproven remedies. **Many patients have been made considerably worse, and many have been made financially bankrupt.** I believe that it is better for patients to understand energy rather than try for instant cures.

Self-help groups
Doctors must understand self-help groups. As with all such organisations, doctors have to be aware of the objects of the group and I have written a chapter on this subject in the 3rd edition of this book. Although some may do harm, the national organisations can be recommended (ME Association, Action for ME). In my experience, **patients have derived great benefit from being a member of a national self-help group** (Ho-Yen DO and Grant A. British Medical Journal 1994; 308: 1298-1299).

PATIENT'S ROLE

When patients are told that they have a major role to play in managing their illness, there is usually disbelief. **They cannot believe that they have to adopt the five steps to better recovery (Figure 33).** Many patients react with "But what about the doctors? After all, it's their job to make me better". Although this is essentially true, in PVFS there is no effective treatment currently available. Management depends upon maintaining the patient's mental attitude, and attempting to alleviate any symptoms that are present. **The traditional medical approach of treatment with drugs and tablets is doomed to failure.** Recovery is best achieved by patients changing their lifestyle to take into account their body's changed capabilities. The doctor's role is secondary – not to treat PVFS, but to ensure that the patient does not have any other treatable illness. In particular, when new symptoms develop, doctors and hospitals are able to provide reassurance that there is no other cause of the symptoms by the use of traditional, diagnostic methods. **Patients, knowing that PVFS is responsible can then start to understand their symptoms and modify their behaviour accordingly.** The role of patients is to understand the media; take responsibility for their illness; and find their own answers to questions.

The Media

Many patients are very influenced by adverse reports in the media. Such articles and programmes are often interpreted as direct criticism by the patient. This emotional reaction is very difficult to deal with and may even cause a relapse. **This is sad and unnecessary. Patients should recognise that the media frequently gets its facts wrong.** When patients see or hear adverse comments, they should not react with anger, horror or disgust. Instead, they should ask the simple question: "Are the facts correct?" If the answer is no, the programme or article should be ignored. If the answer is yes, patients should think again about why their reactions were negative. **A solution is possible for PVFS patients, but patients must first try to assess the media without too**

much emotion.

Many doctors are greatly annoyed at having to deal with upset patients after media attention. It will be a great relief to doctors if patients are able to see these news stories in perspective. One does not go to see one's Member of Parliament after every political story in the media. In the vast majority of cases, the relevance of a political story to the patient's life is the same as a PVFS story. However, **with the hurt of illness, it is easy to get media stories out of perspective.**

Personal Responsibility

Many patients treat PVFS like a bit of sticky tape which they keep trying to throw away. They fail and the tape keeps getting stuck to their clothing and shoes, causing great annoyance. **In fact PVFS is a giant cross which has to be carried.** It is a full time job, requiring all of the patient's resources. It cannot and should not be forgotten that if one is carrying a heavy load, loss of concentration results in a stumble, then a fall.

The medical management of PVFS requires that patients take responsibility for their illness. Patients derive greatest help from themselves (Figure 34). Patients need to adopt a plan and undertake the steps to recovery (Figure 33). It will not be easy. In most cases it will be the most difficult task that they have ever undertaken. **As with many difficulties in life, survival and good health can be great prizes.**

Finding Answers

As every parent knows, children find it easy to ask questions. However, part of the upbringing of children is to teach the children to find answers to their own questions.

224

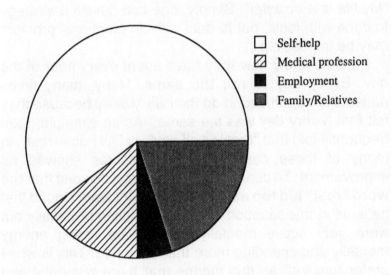

Legend:
- □ Self-help
- ▨ Medical profession
- ■ Employment
- ▨ Family/Relatives

Figure 34   Help in PVFS
Patients obtain greatest help from themselves. Their close family or relatives are next most important. Supportive help provided by the medical profession, and an understanding employer can be a great asset!

Similarly, PVFS patients need to try their own answers to their questions. **Before one is able to find answers to problems, it is necessary to have an accurate assessment of the current position.** Most patients would describe their current position as "a disaster", "chaos", or "grief and mega-grief". Whilst these expressions are colourful, and perhaps true, **it is better to have an assessment that is factual rather than emotional.** Therefore, "I cannot cope with my job" is more useful than "My life is a disaster". Simply, one can devise a strategy to cope with facts, but to deal with an emotional problem may be impossible.

Patients know how they have spent every hour of the day. **Every day is not the same.** Many, many times patients have refused to do their daily diary because they felt that "every day was the same." As an example, I am frequently told that "I rested all day", or "All I do is rest". In many of these cases, the diary scores showed no improvement. To deal with this problem, I decided that **the word "rest" hid too many activities.** Instead, I found that patients in this situation often were resting physically but were very active mentally. They were losing energy mentally and spending more than they had. This is why I prefer "unwind" as this means that there is mental and physical reduction in activities. I like to hear patients say **"I unwind most of the day".**

CONCLUSION

Supportive measures are useful aids for patients. **In all cases, patients should first try to understand energy as this can help all symptoms.** However, for short periods, the medical profession can offer other support. In many cases, the best results will be achieved by trying several medical preparations. Doctors with patience and the will to try different remedies will achieve the best results. Matters will be helped if both patient and doctor can show good humour during this difficult process.

SUMMARY

1. Medical knowledge of PVFS is in its infancy. The syndrome does exist. Cognitive behaviour therapy is helpful, but graded exercise can be harmful. Exercise should increase only when diary scores are 8/10.

2. Better recovery requires a partnership between doctor and patient.

3. The doctor's role in medical assessment involves diagnosis, excluding other diagnoses (Chronic Pain Syndrome, Primary Fibromyalgia Syndrome) and identifying the patient's problems.

4. Medical treatment is supportive. Patients have to be encouraged to help themselves by adopting the five steps to a better recovery. Self-help groups may be of great benefit.

5. Other supportive treatment involves use of pain killers, antidepressants and sleeping tablets. Other measures such as antifungal treatment have more limited application.

6. The patient's role in management involves an understanding of the media, taking personal responsibility for the illness and finding his/her own answers to questions.

CHAPTER FIFTEEN
CONCLUSION

In the late eighties in London, young dealers in the city could make one million pounds for their company before lunch and earn themselves ten thousand pounds commission. They had two bottle lunches and only drank champagne. In the same place, Buddy lived. He was a teenager who had run away from home, did not have a job and lived on the streets. He was regarded as being very simple. The young dealers would pour out onto the pavement after their hundred pound lunches and stop to speak to Buddy. Buddy amused them and made them feel good. They would say:

"Buddy! What would you choose between this shiny metal fifty pence coin and an old paper ten pound note?"

Buddy would always hesitate, he would point a grubby finger at one and then at the other. His eyes would widen and he would always choose the fifty pence coin. The young dealers would laugh and shake their heads in dismay at Buddy's predicament. Sometimes, a group of them would take it in turns to test Buddy. Each day he would perform at least fifty times.

The terrible nineties came and most of the young dealers lost their jobs. One day, one dealer who had been unemployed for two years returned. He saw Buddy, felt remorse and said:

"Buddy, I have to tell you the ten pound paper note is worth more than the shiny metal fifty pence coin."

"Oh yes, I know! But if I choose the ten pound note, I would not get offered the choice again. Anyway, I'm still in work and you are looking for a job."

PVFS patients have to choose less to get more; like Buddy, it is the long-term results that are important. Life is full of divisions: male or female; married or single; employed or unemployed; well or ill. Many PVFS patients feel that their past was full of adventure and good times. Now, they have bad cards. They see their acquaintances, often with less ability (but more energy), doing well and apparently prospering. In comparison, a patient's lot seems to be coming to terms with constant fatigue, intermittent infections, unemployment, separation and divorce. **There seems to be only one major life-event to come – death; and, many wish it soon.**

Patients spend a lot of their time mourning their past existence. They remember times when the sun always shone, when there was frenetic activity and applause. Their current lives appear to be rainy days, pain, discomfort and sadness. **Like all mourning, the whole exercise can take six months.** Sadly, patients are as in Figure 35. They gradually find themselves in the bog of PVFS. Fortunately, there is a path through the bog. **The path is difficult and there are many opportunities for disaster.** Yet, there is also much scope to get more out of life. Anyone can do well when they have unlimited resources. **The real test of ability is to succeed with very limited resources. PVFS patients have very, very limited resources.**

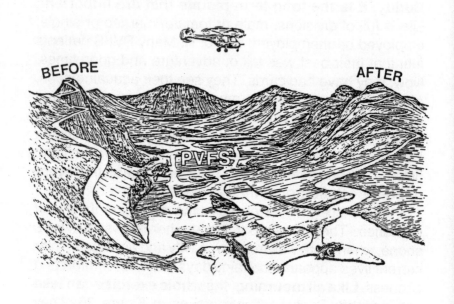

Figure 35 The bog of PVFS
Patients want the medical profession to take them, in a helicopter, from the mountain top before PVFS to the mountain top after PVFS. This helicopter does not exist. Instead, patients gradually slide into the bog of PVFS. But there can be life after PVFS. The way to recovery is there but difficult to find.

FUTURE MEDICAL TREATMENT

With PVFS, the hypothesis is that in a small number of people, during an acute viral infection, there is widespread immunological damage to many tissues. The damage to these tissues takes years to be repaired. In addition, many patients have an immunological system that continues to function abnormally, and this can cause additional damage, thereby further delaying a return to good health. In the next few decades, it is likely that it will be possible to correct the immunological abnormalities that follow the acute infection. **Thus, the continuing damage to the body's tissues will be prevented, and the principal effects of PVFS will be confined to injuries to tissues during the acute viral infection.**

An even more profound effect on patients with PVFS is also possible. In the above hypothesis it is assumed that most of the damage is done at the time of the acute infection. This may be incorrect. **Another suggestion is that the continuing malfunction of the immune system is responsible for the continuing disease.** Thus, the disease can be cured if the immunological abnormalities are corrected. In time, the truth will be known, but whichever hypothesis is correct, medical manipulation of the immune system will be of great help to PVFS patients.

Further decades will also see developments in augmenting the body's ability to repair damaged tissues. Such developments are in the future and are secondary for PVFS patients (i.e. it is far more important to be able to prevent damage than to help with its repair). Prevention is another area in which there is likely to be great change. **In the future, it will be possible to vaccinate susceptible individuals against infections**

associated with PVFS.

In summary, the future outlook for effective medical treatment is very good. It seems very likely that measures will be possible that would allow correction of the abnormalities in PVFS, and more important, protective measures (such as vaccines) will prevent many from developing the illness. Unfortunately, this offers very little comfort for the patient who now has the disease. **At present, for PVFS patients and their medical practitioners there is no easy option.**

A GREAT OPPORTUNITY

It is disastrous when a young, intelligent, extroverted, athletic individual becomes depressed, introverted and somnolent. Many feel that they have no reason for living. Paradoxically, few friends of patients would agree. Indeed patients' acquaintances often have too great an admiration and expectation of patients. The reason for this is that most patients were individuals who got on with living life. However, PVFS does not mean that they should stop living, it only means that they need to change their lifestyle. **It is said that a pessimist is someone who sees disaster in every opportunity, and an optimist is someone who can see opportunity in every disaster.** PVFS patients need to be optimists. They need to hold on to their zest for life.

One great advantage of their condition is that patients have to spend more time in sedentary activities. This leaves a great deal of time for thinking; mental activity uses energy slower than physical activity. Many patients before their illness were so busy living that they had no time to consider what were their life's values, or where they were going. **Energetic activity can be the only reason for living and this occupies most of the non-working hours.**

It is better when exercise is not the only recreational activity. Many sportspersons can find themselves in the position of continuing to play sports because they are good at it, rather than that the activity gives them happiness. Some exercise is necessary for everyone and for those with PVFS it has to be minimal. Instead, these patients have an opportunity to express themselves in other activities. **Many patients can find themselves in new, more enjoyable relationships with this change of lifestyle.** More important, they will have learned that in different stages of life, different patterns of living are more appropriate.

These individuals will also be much happier in the later years of life, as they will have had to come to terms with the frailty of the body early in life. Thus, the limitations of PVFS afford patients the opportunity to consider their talents and abilities, and decide on their life's objectives. Not surprisingly, many patients are much happier with themselves as individuals. This adaptation also has the advantage of preparing one for other changes in life.

ADVANTAGES

Are there any advantages in the patient's situation? What are the "equalizers"? There are two. First is how the patient copes with PVFS. **This is a university, an assault course, a test of survival; graduation and survival will**

ingrain patients with a deep knowledge of themselves. The second is in the patient's potential for happiness. Perhaps, the only equality in the world is each individual's potential for happiness. Each person, no matter how disadvantaged, probably has the same amount of potential for happiness each day as the most privileged. **Happiness is there, it is free; but, many refuse to take their allotted portion, simply because they are ill.** Illness can give patients the understanding that they can be happy if they choose to be – every day.

Life is short. For many, it is a catalogue of lost opportunities. **Patients have to decide if PVFS is a disaster or an opportunity.** The way to better recovery involves personal commitment, hard work, self-understanding and the need for optimism. Very few in the population are given the situation that requires acquisition of such qualities. One should remember that great pressures, over many years, are required to make a diamond – the hardest of all minerals, able to withstand much stress.

A PVFS patient has a terrible affliction at the wrong time of life. Yet, coping with the illness and its consequences produces a very special person: one capable of coping with strife, but able to enjoy the sunshine between the storms.

INDEX

Unwind!

Understand and control life, be better!!

(ISBN 0-9511090-2-2)

by Dr Darrel Ho-Yen

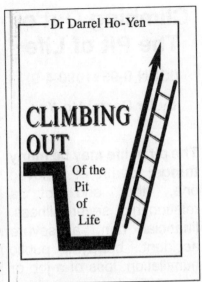

Dr Darrel Ho-Yen

CLIMBING OUT

Of the Pit of Life

Many individuals are having great difficulties in living in a modern society. The stress on these people may produce ill health. This book shows that stress can be reduced by the acquisition of skills. **This book was first published in 1991 and reprinted in 1994.**

The skill of unwinding (EMBME) is explained in great detail and has benefits of physical and mental relaxation. **Both well and ill individuals would benefit from this skill.**

With the ability to unwind, you can start to develop an understanding of your life and identify your own problems. Control of your life is achieved by good use of time, use of the reward/effort ratio and good decision-making. **With the acquisition of these skills, you have the opportunity for self-improvement, happiness and to be better.**

Obtainable from: Dodona Books

Climbing Out of The Pit of Life

(ISBN 0-9511090-4-9)

by Dr Darrel Ho-Yen

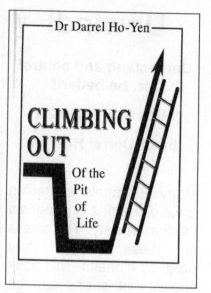

The pit of life may be many things: death of a loved one, the end of a relationship, severe illness, financial ruin, a severe accident, betrayal, public humiliation, loss of a job or an enforced change of life.

How do some people recovery quickly whilst others may never recovery? How does one cope with these crises? The ladder (**l**ifeless, **a**nger, **d**enial, **d**isgrace, **e**ndeavour, **r**enewal) describes the stages one needs to go through to cope with great loss.

Dr Ho-Yen describes in details what one suffers and offers clear, practical solutions to each problem. It empowers the individual to recovery quickly

Obtainable from Dodona Books